A Woman's Guide to
Pelvic Health

A Woman's Guide to

PELVIC HEALTH

Expert Advice for Women of All Ages

ELIZABETH E. HOUSER, M.D.
and
STEPHANIE RILEY HAHN, P.T.

THE JOHNS HOPKINS
UNIVERSITY PRESS
Baltimore

Note to the Reader: The information in this book should by no means be considered a substitute for the advice of qualified medical professionals. The descriptions and illustrations of women's pelvic problems provided in this book are examples only. A person may have pelvic problems that do not look like or act like any of the examples in this book. If you are worried about any pelvic symptoms, you need to consult a qualified medical professional. An examination with a qualified medical professional is recommended at least once a year. The services of a competent professional should be obtained whenever medical or other specific advice is needed.

All efforts have been made to ensure the accuracy of the information contained in this book as of the date of publication. The author and the publisher expressly disclaim responsibility for any adverse outcomes arising from the use or application of the information contained herein.

© 2012 Elizabeth E. Houser and Stephanie Riley Hahn
All rights reserved. Published 2012
Printed in the United States of America on acid-free paper
9 8 7 6 5 4 3 2 1

The Johns Hopkins University Press
2715 North Charles Street
Baltimore, Maryland 21218-4363
www.press.jhu.edu

Library of Congress Cataloging-in-Publication Data
Houser, Elizabeth E.
    A woman's guide to pelvic health : expert advice for women of all ages /
Elizabeth E. Houser and Stephanie Riley Hahn.
        p. cm.
    Includes bibliographical references and index.
    ISBN 978-1-4214-0691-6 (hdbk. : alk. paper) — ISBN 978-1-4214-0692-3 (pbk. : alk. paper) — ISBN 978-1-4214-0757-9 (electronic) — ISBN 1-4214-0691-8 (hdbk. : alk. paper) — ISBN 1-4214-0692-6 (pbk. : alk. paper) — ISBN 1-4214-0757-4 (electronic)
    1. Pelvic floor—Diseases—Popular works.   2. Pelvic floor—Diseases—Treatment—Popular works.   3. Urinary incontinence—Physical therapy—Popular works.
4. Women—Health and hygiene—Popular works.   5. Self-care, Health—Popular works.   I. Hahn, Stephanie Riley.   II. Title.
    RG482.H68 2013
    616.6'20082—dc23   2012008905

A catalog record for this book is available from the British Library.

Figures 1.1, 1.2, 1.3, 2.1, 3.1, 5.1, 5.2, 7.1, 7.4, 7.5, and 7.8 are by Mary Crisler.
Figures 7.2, 7.3, 7.6, 7.7, 7.9, 7.10, 7.11, and 7.12 are by Holly Williams Photography.

Special discounts are available for bulk purchases of this book. For more information, please contact Special Sales at 410-516-6936 or specialsales@press.jhu.edu.

The Johns Hopkins University Press uses environmentally friendly book materials, including recycled text paper that is composed of at least 30 percent postconsumer waste, whenever possible.

To all women who need help with their pelvic disorders

Contents

Foreword

Millions of women begrudgingly toss adult diapers or feminine pads into their grocery carts each week, unaware that effective solutions are available to treat their leaking bladders. As a family physician, I know that many of my patients are embarrassed to talk about their symptoms, even when I raise the topic. Women often believe that major surgery is the only option. Most have never even heard of physical therapy for issues such as urinary or sexual problems.

Urologist Elizabeth Houser and physical therapist Stephanie Hahn have 33 years of combined clinical experience directly helping thousands of women overcome bladder and sexual dysfunctions. This book provides answers to questions that many women are too nervous or embarrassed to ask their doctors.

The authors clearly explain how weakened pelvic floor muscles— as a result of childbirth, aging, or other lifestyle issues—can lead to distressing symptoms such as urinary incontinence. Each condition is covered individually, with detailed and easily understood descriptions. *In the privacy of their homes*, women with pelvic floor disorders can learn about the specific symptoms of their condition, medical tests to confirm their diagnosis, and myriad treatment options, from Kegels or acupuncture to medication or surgery. Side effects and success rates for each treatment option are discussed, as well as ways women can ask their doctors for help. The detailed at-home pelvic floor retraining program offers women a chance to alleviate symptoms on their own, step by step and week by week. This book is a practical guide delivered with compassion and understanding.

Women must seek help sooner rather than later since the probability of symptom improvement decreases over time, and conservative approaches, which may help some women avoid surgery, are more effective when used soon after symptoms occur. This book will give readers the confidence and knowledge to successfully address their bladder and sexual concerns with their health care providers, plus the tools to immediately begin a home program.

You need not be doomed to decades of accidents and extra laundry. The compassionate, practical information packed in this book will help you start jogging down that road to a healthier, drier you.

Jill Grimes, M.D.

Family Physician and Author of *Seductive Delusions:*
How Everyday People Catch STDs

www.JillGrimesMD.com

Associate Editor, *5-Minute Clinical Consult—*
Medical Professionals' Leading Choice for Trusted
Clinical Content

Acknowledgments

Thanks go out to all the women in our urology and physical therapy practices who showed us how best to help them with their pelvic disorders; their requests paved the way for the content in this book. We want to thank our editor, Stephanie Yeh, who partnered with us from the start to turn our passion into this completed project. Thanks also go to our agent, Jeanne Fredericks, who worked tirelessly to find a home for this book. We are grateful to Johns Hopkins University Press executive editor Jacqueline Wehmueller and to editorial assistant Sara Cleary, who have made this process so smooth. We want to thank Mary Crisler for her ability to turn ideas into incredible illustrations. Our gratitude goes to Holly Williams for her beautiful photography and to Natalie Gauci, our model. Last but not least, we thank our friend and cheerleader Jill Grimes, who helped us immensely with the logistics of this book.

I WANT TO THANK MY HUSBAND, Chuck, who supported me while I laughed and cried writing this book. I also want to express my deep gratitude to my parents, Edward and Kay Houser, and my siblings, Melissa and Bruce Houser, who taught me to pursue my dreams without reservation. Thanks also go out to my extended family and friends, who acted as both cheerleaders and sounding boards throughout this whole process. Special thanks to my colleagues and mentors, Shelley Green, Douglas Flemons, Melody Denson, George Webster, and Jill

Grimes, who have all inspired me to share my medical experiences and expertise with women in need. I will not forget the hundreds of women who have entrusted me with their most private, pelvic health—this book is for you. Finally, I especially thank my partner in this book, Stephanie Hahn, who brought her depth of knowledge of pelvic floor anatomy and function to this book. Without her partnership, this book would not be complete.

Elizabeth E. Houser, M.D.

I WANT TO FIRST ACKNOWLEDGE GOD for giving me the unique talents and interest I have for helping women with pelvic floor disorders to heal and recover a more active lifestyle. Thank you to my extremely supportive and loving husband, Michael, who first experienced my anguish at becoming incontinent at the age of 30 with a brand-new son. Michael has championed me these last 16 years as I have continued this journey both personally and professionally. I want to acknowledge my three sons for their understanding and encouragement during the three-plus years of writing this book. Next, thanks go to my parents, Bob and Peggy Riley, for instilling in me the desire to set and reach a goal that will enrich the lives of others around me. My gratitude goes to Mark Strickland and Resa Meinholdt, who both believed in the need for physical therapy to help address pelvic floor disorders and who offered support as we opened the first physical therapy practice in Austin, Texas, to focus on women's health issues. Thanks to Diana Feltz, my mentor and friend, who taught me the art of Pilates. For my many patients and Pilates clients, who over the years have taught me how to help others, this book is for you. Thank you to my amazing friend and book partner, Elizabeth Houser, who has shared with me her passion and knowledge, and so much more, during these many years. Finally, to my extended family and friends, who have been encouraging and praying for me as I have walked this path, thank you!

Stephanie Riley Hahn, P.T.

A Woman's Guide to
Pelvic Health

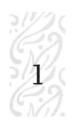

1

Anatomy and Pelvic Floor Health

Is This You?

JANE, IN HER MID-THIRTIES, loves how kickboxing is helping restore her figure after she gave birth to her adorable son. What she doesn't love is the amount of urine she leaks every time she kicks or boxes. In fact, the leakage happens so often that she is thinking of stopping her exercise program altogether.

Here's what Jane doesn't know: She has stress urinary incontinence (also called stress incontinence), the most common form of urinary incontinence, which affects 26 percent of women over age 18 at some point in their lives. Childbirth is a major cause of stress incontinence. Most women with urine leakage wait more than six years to get help. Yet research shows that urinary incontinence in 8 out of 10 women with the condition can be improved. How long will Jane wait?

SIXTY-TWO-YEAR-OLD KAREN has bathrooms on the brain. She has to urinate 10 to 12 times a day and a few times at night. Sometimes she feels a sudden urge and doesn't make it to the bathroom in time—she then leaks a large volume of urine. Karen has to carry several changes of clothing with her and buys adult diapers in bulk. Her situation is bad, but her embarrassment about seeking help is worse, so she just keeps coping with the condition by herself.

This is what Karen should know: Karen is suffering from the most severe form of overactive bladder, called urge urinary incontinence. About 17 percent of women in the United States have urge incontinence, especially women 50 and older, but less than half seek help. Getting help is important, because about 60 percent of women with urge urinary incontinence also experience depression (though the two conditions are not always related). Help is also important because 70 percent of women with urge incontinence report symptom improvement with conservative treatments like medication or physical therapy.

JO, AGE 40 AND VERY FIT, faces a complex situation: she has the same symptoms as Jane *and* Karen, meaning she leaks urine when she exercises or laughs as well as because of sudden urges. She's had symptoms for only 11 months but is definitely going to ask her doctor for help, even though she feels embarrassed. Her symptoms are frequent and serious.

What Jo will learn when she talks to her doctor: Jo's doctor will tell her that she has mixed urinary incontinence, which is a combination of stress incontinence *and* urge incontinence or overactive bladder. Women with this mixed form of incontinence are more likely to seek help earlier because their symptoms tend to be worse and more frequent than symptoms of women who experience only stress *or* urge incontinence/overactive bladder. Mixed incontinence has a much stronger negative effect on quality of life, and women with this condition spend much more on laundry bills and adult diapers.

AT AGE 68, SUSAN is suddenly experiencing low-back pain, chronic constipation, and the feeling that she is sitting on a ball. Luckily, she already has an appointment with her ob-gyn in a few weeks. She hopes her doctor will tell her what's happening in her pelvic region.

What Susan's ob-gyn will tell her at her appointment: Susan feels like she's sitting on a ball because her pelvic organs have literally popped out of place. She has pelvic organ prolapse, in which one or more of her pelvic organs have moved out of place and now bulge into other organs. Susan's ob-gyn will tell her that she is among the 3 to 6 percent of women who have severe pelvic organ prolapse, and will most likely need surgery to correct the problem. Surprisingly, between 43 and 76 percent of women have some degree of prolapse without knowing it and should be taking preventive action.

AT AGE 32 CHERIE is supposed to be in her sexual prime, at least according to the latest women's magazines, but she feels far from sexy. With two children and a busy career, she considers sex to be at the bottom of her list. Further, sex with her husband just isn't very pleasurable anymore because Cherie doesn't feel much sensation in her sexual organs. She avoids sex as much as possible, but her husband is becoming upset and worried. She knows she needs to do something to resolve the situation, but she doesn't know what.

How Cherie can solve her sexual problem: More than 40 percent of women are dissatisfied with their sex lives, and many of these women have decreased sexual sensation, which is what Cherie is experiencing. This decrease in sensation is often due to weak pelvic floor muscles, and the good news is that these muscles can easily be strengthened with pelvic floor muscle exercises. Studies show that women who do pelvic floor exercises reach orgasm more easily and experience more sexual desire. Cherie can improve her symptoms by following a simple pelvic floor exercise program, such as one from her physical therapist or the at-home program in chapter 7 of this book.

What's Happening with Your Pelvic Floor?

If you relate to any of the women's experiences described in the previous pages, then you probably want to know what is happening with your pelvic floor. The quiz in this chapter, along with the rest of the chapters in this book, will provide you with the information you need. This book covers five conditions associated with the pelvic floor:

1. Stress urinary incontinence
2. Overactive bladder, including urge urinary incontinence

3. Mixed urinary incontinence—a combination of stress and urge incontinence or overactive bladder
4. Pelvic organ prolapse
5. Decreased sexual sensation

Reading the chapters about each of these conditions will give you a good idea of the related symptoms and the facts you need to know about each condition, including treatment options.

To get a quick idea of which condition or conditions may be affecting your quality of life, take our simple Pelvic Floor IQ quiz in the following section. Once you have completed the test and calculated your results, you will have a good idea of which chapters to read first. Although the test is only a guideline and not a definitive diagnosis of your condition, it will give you solid insight into what is happening with your pelvic floor.

What Is Your Pelvic Floor IQ?

To discover what is going on with your pelvic floor, read each question in table 1.1, on page 6. Place a check mark next to each question to which you answer "Yes." After you have completed all the questions, follow the instructions at the top of the quiz to calculate your results. Write these results in table 1.2.

To translate your results from the test, refer to this key:

S = Stress urinary incontinence
O = Overactive bladder / urge urinary incontinence
P = Pelvic organ prolapse
D = Decreased sexual sensation

If you scored a 2 or higher for any of the conditions, then you may be experiencing those conditions. If you have scored a 2 or higher for both S and O categories, you may have a condition called mixed urinary incontinence, which is a combination of stress urinary incontinence and overactive bladder or urge urinary incontinence. If so, you'll want to read the chapters associated with all three conditions. The chapters related to each pelvic floor condition discussed in this book are:

Chapter 2: Stress urinary incontinence
Chapter 3: Overactive bladder and urge urinary incontinence
Chapter 4: Mixed urinary incontinence
Chapter 5: Pelvic organ prolapse
Chapter 6: Decreased sexual sensation

Now that you have a better idea of what is happening with your pelvis, you can read and learn about the conditions that may be affecting you and your quality of life. You will be taking the first step toward improving your condition.

Prepare to say goodbye to embarrassing symptoms, quiet suffering, coping mechanisms, and a limited lifestyle. We encourage you to welcome a new sense of freedom into your life. Start by learning more about your pelvic anatomy and how it works by reading the rest of this chapter. A little knowledge of anatomy will go a long way toward understanding your condition. Then dive into the chapters that are most relevant to you, as well as chapter 7, which describes an effective at-home pelvic floor exercise program you can use to improve or even cure your symptoms.

A note about intrinsic sphincter deficiency and overflow incontinence

Two other types of incontinence deserve mention. Intrinsic sphincter deficiency (ISD) occurs when the closure pressure of the urethral sphincter is lower than the bladder pressure. In other words, the pelvic floor muscles that normally prevent leakage are weak. Although ISD can occur with prolapse of the bladder (cystocele), the rectum or large bowel (rectocele), or the small intestine or small bowel (enterocele), the prolapse is usually not severe.[1] ISD often occurs in elderly women because the urethra thins after menopause. For this reason, the condition can be treated with bulking agents injected around the urethra or with

TABLE 1.1 Pelvic Floor IQ quiz

Count the total number of check marks associated with each letter (S, O, P, D) and list the totals in table 1.2.

	Check if "Yes"
1. Do you leak urine when you clear your throat, cough, sneeze, or laugh?	_____ S
2. Do you wake up two or more times during the night to urinate?	_____ O
3. Do you feel sudden urges to urinate whether or not you experience urine leakage?	_____ O
4. Do you have difficulty reaching orgasm during sex?	_____ D
5. Do you feel pulling, stretching, or pressure in your low back or groin?	_____ P
6. Have you experienced less sexual satisfaction or sensation in your sexual organs after menopause?	_____ D
7. Do you see a bulge pushing out of your vagina or feel as if something is falling out of your vagina?	_____ P
8. Do you have less sensation than you used to in your sexual organs?	_____ D
9. Do you leak urine when stepping up or down, or changing position?	_____ S
10. Do you feel the need to urinate eight or more times daily or shortly after you have emptied your bladder?	_____ O
11. Do you experience urine leakage when lifting something?	_____ S
12. Do you feel little or no sensation in your sexual organs during sex (including masturbation)?	_____ D
13. Do you have urinary incontinence during physical exercise?	_____ S
14. Do you experience painful sex?	_____ P
15. Do you experience the urge to urinate when you hear the sound of running water?	_____ O
16. Do you have constipation or difficult urination improved by pressing your fingers into your abdomen or vagina?	_____ P
17. Do you have urine leakage when engaging in physical activities of any kind?	_____ S
18. Do you have little or no interest in sex because you do not feel pleasurable sensations during sex?	_____ D
19. Do you have strong urges to urinate after drinking small amounts of water, or after eating or drinking certain foods or beverages?	_____ O
20. Do you feel the pressure of pelvic organs pushing into your vagina or do you feel as if you are sitting on a ball?	_____ P

S = Stress urinary incontinence; O = Overactive bladder / urge urinary incontinence; P = Pelvic organ prolapse; D = Decreased sexual sensation

TABLE 1.2   Pelvic Floor IQ quiz results

In the table below, list your totals for each letter from table 1.1.

S	O	P	D

S = Stress urinary incontinence; O = Overactive bladder/urge urinary incontinence;
P = Pelvic organ prolapse; D = Decreased sexual sensation

the surgical placement of a tape or sling. Transvaginal estrogen, in the form of a cream, tablet, or ring, works well, as does a pessary.

Overflow incontinence occurs when the bladder cannot empty completely, so that the pressure in the bladder becomes high enough to overcome the urethral pressure. This condition is common in patients with neurological diseases or diabetes. Overflow incontinence can be treated with self-catheterization several times a day, a procedure that your doctor can teach you to do. Another option for treating overflow incontinence is sacral neuromodulation, which involves an implantable device that stimulates the nerves to the bladder. As we discuss in chapter 3, this device is implanted in the buttock, under the skin, and has a thin lead wire that is anchored near the sacral nerve and runs through the tailbone. The lead can be programmed to help a woman fully void her bladder and later be reprogrammed to allow her to void on her own. This device is also approved for urinary retention, urge incontinence that does not respond to medication, urinary frequency, and general urinary incontinence.

Meet Your Pelvic Floor

Don't worry. We won't bore you with mind-boggling scientific terms or complicated diagrams. Instead, we provide a simple introduction to your pelvic region. With a basic understanding of your pelvic anatomy, you will be better able to comprehend the information given in later chapters, including what's causing your condition, diagnostic tests your doctor might perform, and the science behind conservative and surgical treatment options.

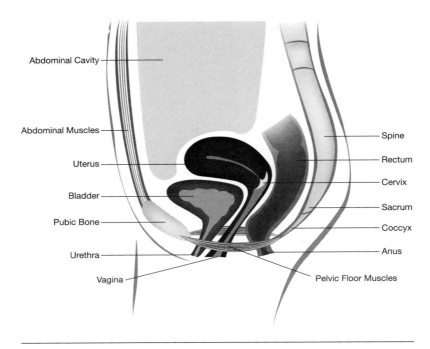

Labels on figure:
- Abdominal Cavity
- Abdominal Muscles
- Uterus
- Bladder
- Pubic Bone
- Urethra
- Vagina
- Spine
- Rectum
- Cervix
- Sacrum
- Coccyx
- Anus
- Pelvic Floor Muscles

FIGURE 1.1. Basic view of pelvic anatomy

Let's begin with the pelvic floor, which is not only the basis of this book but also the literal foundation of your pelvic health. "Pelvic floor" can be a confusing term. For our purposes, we refer to the pelvic floor muscles as the collection of all muscles found in the base of the pelvis between the pubic bone, at the front of your pelvis, and the coccyx, or the tip of the tailbone.

Visualize your pelvis as a bowl, with the pelvic floor muscles forming a hammock that covers the bottom of that bowl. This hammock is connected to the pubic bone in front and the coccyx in back, and it is connected side to side to different pelvic bones. There are three openings in your pelvic floor muscles: the urethra, vagina, and anus. This sheet of muscles supports your pelvic organs, including your vagina, bladder, urethra, and rectum. See figure 1.1 for a basic view of pelvic anatomy.

The pelvic floor muscles are composed of both superficial and deep muscle layers. The superficial muscles, shown in lighter shading in figure 1.2, are closer to the skin and assist with clitoral erection and tightening of the vaginal sphincter. Both are important to pleasurable sexual sensation. These muscles also help support the perineum, the area between the vagina and anus, when abdominal pressure increases. This support prevents urinary leakage when you sneeze or cough. Additional muscles in this superficial layer (deep transverse perineal muscle and anal sphincter) also assist in tightening the sphincters. The deeper muscle layers are located more internally. Shown in the darkest shading in figure 1.2, these muscles act as sphincters for all three pelvic openings (urethra, vagina, and anus), contracting and relaxing these openings as needed. The deeper muscles also support the contents of the pelvis as well as the pelvic bones and joints.

Collectively, the pelvic floor muscles assist in supporting the pelvic organs against the effects of gravity, provide sphincter control to withstand external forces on the bladder and rectum, and aid in increasing sexual response. Healthy pelvic floor muscles work together as a dynamic elastic system that responds to your body's changing needs. For instance, when you sneeze, and your intra-abdominal pressure increases, these muscles should contract to keep waste from exiting the bladder and bowels. When you need to urinate and your bladder contracts, your pelvic floor muscles should relax to allow urine to exit your body. When your body is at rest, these muscles support your pelvic organs and prevent them from sagging out of place. Last, the friction caused by strong pelvic floor muscles aids in female arousal, because the nerve endings in these muscles provide resistance to a penetrating penis. There are few nerve endings in the vaginal canal, so women don't experience much arousal from vaginal penetration.

Within these pelvic muscles, scientists have identified both Type I and Type II motor fibers. The Type I motor fibers, also called "slow twitch" muscle fibers, are responsible for long, enduring support within the pelvis. The Type II fibers, on the other hand, are called "fast twitch" fibers and are responsible for rapid reactive sphincter compression, which is what prevents urine leakage during a sneeze

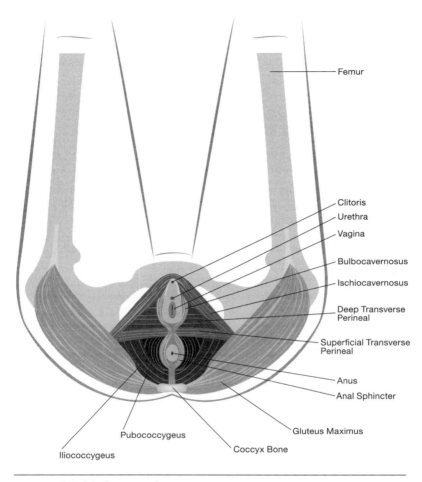

FIGURE 1.2. Pelvic floor muscles

or cough. The at-home pelvic floor program in chapter 7, which helps you develop pelvic floor muscle strength and endurance, trains both types of muscle fibers.

The anatomy of the urinary system

The components of your urinary system, shown in figure 1.3, are just as important as the pelvic floor muscles. These components work

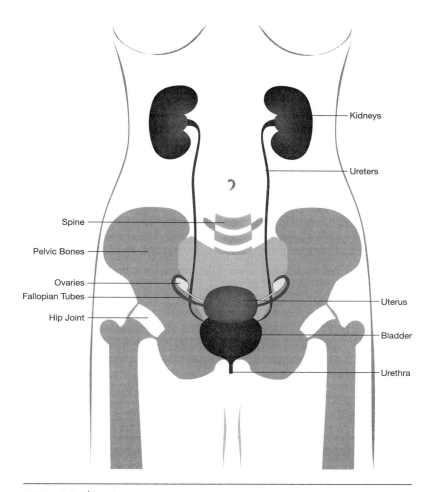

FIGURE 1.3. The urinary system

together as a synchronized waste-removal system. First, the kidneys produce urine by filtering excess water and waste products from the bloodstream. The urine is carried from the kidneys to the bladder by tubes called ureters.

The bladder, which is a hollow muscular organ that sits in the pelvis, receives and stores the urine until you are ready to urinate. The bladder is held in place by ligaments attached to other pelvic organs and to the pelvic bones. As urine accumulates, the bladder swells into a round balloon-like shape. A healthy bladder can store up to 16 ounces (two cups) of urine comfortably for two to five hours. As the bladder fills with urine, circular muscles called sphincters close tightly to keep urine in the bladder. When your bladder becomes full, nerves in your bladder will send signals to your brain, and you will feel the urge to urinate.

When you are ready to urinate, your brain signals the urinary sphincters to relax and the bladder to contract, squeezing urine out of the bladder and into the urethra. Urine can then leave the bladder through the urethra. When these signals occur in the correct order, normal urination occurs. When these signals get mixed up, you experience urinary incontinence and other symptoms. Luckily, with the techniques and treatment options we offer in this book, you can "retrain" your bladder and brain, as well as adjust your lifestyle habits to prevent incontinence.

Now that you have an understanding of your basic pelvic anatomy, it is time to learn the specifics of your condition . . . and what you can do to improve the quality of your life.

2

Stress Urinary Incontinence

MY STORY:
Recovery from Stress Urinary Incontinence

After having two delightful daughters by natural deliveries, I was thrilled with the birth of my son—another joyous event. What didn't thrill me was an unexpected post-delivery health issue. I suffered daily from urinary incontinence, which had not occurred after the births of my daughters. This meant that I leaked urine every time I picked up my son, stepped off a curb, or sneezed. Despite my two prior vaginal deliveries, nothing like this had ever happened to me. I had always been quite healthy.

After each baby I had returned to exercising to regain my pre-pregnancy weight. When I tried to do this after the birth of my son, I had to cope with the urine leakage by using pads or carrying changes of clothes around. I finally realized that the situation was so bad that I had to get help from my doctor. After all, I was only 36 years old.

I was relieved when my doctor told me that my pelvic organs were still in good position. I had stress urinary incontinence, which meant I leaked urine anytime I put pressure on my bladder. My pelvic muscle tone was decreased from the pregnancy and the stress of my third vaginal delivery. When she asked me to do a Kegel (pelvic floor muscle contraction) during the exam, I contracted my buttock muscles instead of the muscles in my pelvic floor, which meant that my Kegels weren't doing anything to control the urinary leakage. I found out that my condition could probably be treated with conservative measures like physical therapy. Apparently, my insurance company agreed, because they authorized eight sessions with a physical therapist specializing in pelvic floor rehabilitation.

I faithfully attended physical therapy sessions and was happy to find that my physical therapist was extremely empathetic and professional, especially when it came to the "hands-on" portion of the therapy. She used various methods to help me strengthen my pelvic floor muscles and do correct Kegels. I also learned to retrain my bladder with scheduled bathroom visits and relaxation techniques. My physical therapist and I laughed about the fact that my son and I were doing our potty training together!

Three months later, having done hundreds of Kegels, I felt like I had regained control of my bladder. I was able to prevent the leakage that used to occur daily and could leave the house without having to carry pads or extra clothes with me. I did Kegels any time I picked up my son or had to sneeze, and I experienced no urine leakage accidents. Strengthening my pelvic floor made an amazing difference in my life, and I will be doing Kegels for the rest of my life. My doctor also shared information about medications that could help if I felt a need to "fine-tune" my bladder control.

Conservative therapies helped me control my urinary incontinence for more than five years, but I eventually started leaking urine again, so I went back to my doctor. I had put on about 15 pounds, and apparently my weight gain plus the effects of aging had stressed my pelvic floor muscles so that Kegels were no longer sufficient to control the incontinence. My doctor suggested a minimally invasive surgery called transobturator tape, in which a mesh tape would be placed around my urethra to prevent leakage. She assured me that it was a simple outpatient procedure.

I wasn't keen to "go under the knife," but I didn't want to deal with daily urine leakage either, so I decided to go ahead with the surgery. Thankfully my doctor was right, and the surgery was quite painless. By following the easy aftercare instructions, I was back to my regular exercise program and busy life routine—with no urine leakage—in less than eight weeks. My doctor encouraged me to keep doing my Kegels and assured me that the transobturator tape surgery would keep me dry for a long time to come.

Stress Urinary Incontinence: No Laughing Matter

The old adage tells us that laughter is the best medicine. But for the woman suffering from stress incontinence, laughter can cause urine leakage, creating embarrassing situations. People with this condition are often afraid not just to laugh, but also to sneeze, lift heavy objects, exercise . . . or do anything at all.

Does that sound like you? If so, you are not alone. Recent studies reveal that urinary incontinence affects more than 30 million American adults, with stress incontinence being the most common form.[1] The National Association for Continence, an advocacy organization dedicated to helping consumers affected by incontinence, offers some startling statistics about urinary incontinence in general:[2]

- Consumer research reveals that one in four women over the age of 18 experiences episodes of leaking urine involuntarily.
- One-third of men and women ages 30 to 70 have experienced loss of bladder control at some point in their adult lives and may still be living with the symptoms.
- On average, women wait six and a half years from the first time they experience symptoms until they obtain a diagnosis for their bladder control problems.
- Two-thirds of individuals who experience loss of bladder control do not use any treatment or product to manage their incontinence.

Unfortunately, as you can probably imagine, most of the people who make up these statistics are too embarrassed to discuss their condition with their doctor. And who wouldn't be? After all, most of us thought we were done with diapers and bladder training when we grew out of toddlerhood. Yet, stress urinary incontinence is a treatable condition, so it's well worth any embarrassment you might experience while talking to your doctor. Later in this chapter, we discuss various ways you can talk to your health care provider and find the right treatment for your situation. Understanding and seeking the right treatment for this type of urinary incontinence can help you avoid socially awkward moments and can make it possible for you to resume activities you enjoy, such as exercising and laughing (not to mention sex).

Treatment can also keep you away from a vicious cycle of weight gain and depression. For instance, if you can't jog or exercise because you leak urine when you do, you may find yourself becoming lethargic, feeling depressed, and slipping into emotional eating patterns. The more you eat, the more weight you gain . . . and naturally the more depressed you become. Shopping for pads and diapers, and repeatedly taking your clothes to the dry cleaners, doesn't help your mental state, not to mention your checkbook. The medical, social, emotional, and financial implications of stress incontinence are huge—and personal. You get the picture. In fact, you may be living this picture, which is why finding the right treatment for you (and we feel we have insight into some particularly effective treatments) is so important.

Ouch! The high cost of urinary incontinence

So what does urinary incontinence really cost you? If you've never sat down with your checkbook and a calculator, you might be surprised. The cost could be higher than you think. One study showed that, on average, women with urinary incontinence spent more than $1,000 per year on diapers, pads, and laundry to manage their condition yet still experienced a significant decrease in their quality of life. This figure does not include nongeneric drug costs, which can exceed $1,300 per year. The study also revealed that the same women were willing to spend up to $1,400 per year for a cure.[3]

Add those individual out-of-pocket expenses to the institutional costs at a national level (such as nursing home costs, UTI treatment, bedsores, catheter-related problems, and so on) and the high price of incontinence is truly alarming. In 2008, the cost of urinary incontinence in the United States was a staggering $19 billion.[4] If that number doesn't shock you—and it should—just think about what will happen as, in coming years, aging baby boomers reach their sixties, seventies, eighties, and beyond.

Urinary incontinence is nothing to laugh about. But don't worry. With our step-by-step pelvic floor rehabilitation program for treating urinary incontinence, you will likely regain your quality of life and save yourself, and the U.S. health care system, a lot of money.

The good news about stress urinary incontinence

These days, there is a lot of good news for women coping with this kind of urinary incontinence. For instance, physicians are becoming much more aware of the problem and are more likely to ask you about and help you with your stress incontinence. According to the American Academy of Family Physicians, urinary incontinence has become a more prevalent issue than even diabetes or asthma for primary care physicians.[5]

Also, a whole array of solutions exists, ranging from conservative to aggressive, depending on your specific situation. Here are some of the treatments that are helping many women with stress urinary incontinence to stay dry:

- Physical therapy and biofeedback
- Medication
- Diet and lifestyle changes
- Acupuncture
- Surgery

Relieving your stress urinary incontinence symptoms may be easier than you think. Did you know that if you are overweight, losing even a few pounds, as little as 5 percent of your body weight, can significantly improve symptoms of your urine leakage?[6] No kidding. If you weigh 150 pounds, for example, and lose 7 or 8 pounds, you may notice a difference.

With so many solutions available, don't waste another moment dealing with urine leakage. Get the help you need. First, read further to learn more about this type of incontinence and what you can do about it. Then, read about and start using our step-by-step pelvic floor retraining system, detailed in chapter 7. This program helps you test the tone of your pelvic floor muscles and teaches you how to strengthen them. Finally, pick up the phone and make an appointment with your doctor. There are so many solutions for stress incontinence, and so few reasons not to ask for help.

What You Need to Know about Stress Urinary Incontinence

What exactly is stress urinary incontinence?

As the name suggests, stress urinary incontinence is a condition that causes you to leak urine anytime you put stress on your abdominal cavity, such as when you cough, sneeze, laugh, jump, or exercise. Just standing up or stepping off a curb can cause leakage, which can be discouraging to even the most optimistic of women. Basically, this type of leakage occurs whenever your intra-abdominal pressure suddenly increases.

How common is stress urinary incontinence?

Recent studies show that 26 percent of women over the age of 18 have experienced this type of urinary incontinence. Experts estimate that general urinary incontinence affects 18 million women in the United States. Specifically, it affects 33 percent of women ages 45 to 64, and 24 percent of women ages 25 to 44.[7] Sixty percent of women who experience urinary incontinence have this type, which is the most common form of incontinence.

What causes stress urinary incontinence?

Stress urinary incontinence happens when the pelvic floor muscles that support the bladder and urethra are weak, or because one of the urethral sphincters, which normally keeps urine from leaking, isn't as strong as it should be.

In women, the main causes of these weakened muscles are the effects of the three G's: gravity, giving birth, and graying (aging). Childbirth, especially multiple childbirths, can cause tears or stretching in the pelvic muscles, or even nerve damage, resulting in weakness. In mild cases, these muscles do not properly support the bladder and urethra, and the sphincter isn't strong enough to stop the flow of urine (see the comparison between a normal bladder and a stress urinary incontinence bladder in figures 2.1a and 2.1b). If your condition is not severe, conservative therapy, which we cover later in this chapter, can resolve your urine leakage symptoms.

In more drastic cases, childbirth can cause what is called pelvic organ prolapse, which literally means that certain pelvic organs bulge into other organs. For instance, the bladder can prolapse and bulge into the vaginal wall; the rectum can also prolapse into the vaginal wall; the small intestine can slip down between the rectum and vagina; and the uterus can drop down into the vagina. Each of these different "bulges" can contribute to stress incontinence and often have to be corrected with surgery.

How do I know if I have stress urinary incontinence?

You know you have stress incontinence if you involuntarily leak urine when you put stress on your bladder by coughing, sneezing, standing, exercising, or engaging in any physical activity.

What are the risk factors for stress urinary incontinence?

The risk factors for this type of urinary incontinence include:

- Being female (twice as many women as men have stress incontinence)
- Childbirth
- Chronic coughing (such as chronic bronchitis or asthma)
- Aging
- Obesity
- Diabetes
- Steroid use
- Smoking

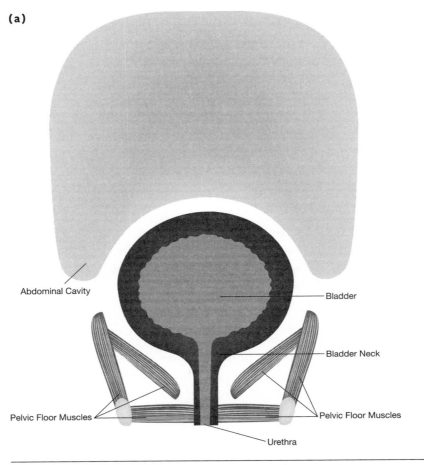

Abdominal Cavity

Bladder

Bladder Neck

Pelvic Floor Muscles

Pelvic Floor Muscles

Urethra

FIGURE 2.1. (a) Healthy bladder. (b) Stress urinary incontinence bladder.

When should I contact a doctor about stress urinary incontinence?

As soon as you notice symptoms of stress incontinence, bring them to the attention of your doctor. As noted earlier in this chapter, doctors are becoming more aware of how common urinary incontinence is, so don't be embarrassed to raise the subject. In fact, the sooner you

(b)

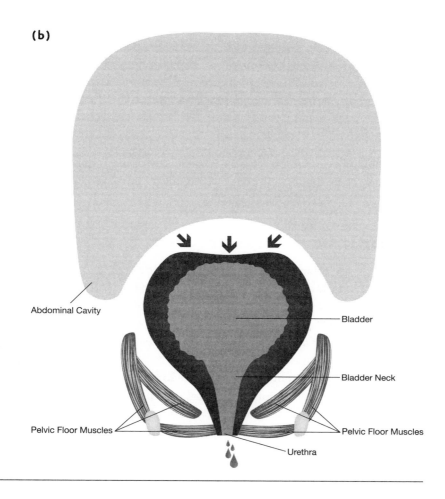

Abdominal Cavity

Bladder

Bladder Neck

Pelvic Floor Muscles

Pelvic Floor Muscles

Urethra

begin treating your urinary incontinence, the more likely you are to experience success with conservative treatments.[8]

In addition, seeking treatment early makes good financial sense, since untreated urinary incontinence can cost upwards of $1,000 per year in adult diapers and laundry bills.[9] Most of the time, your primary care physician will refer you to a specialist, who might be a urologist, urogynecologist, nurse, nurse practitioner, physical therapist, geriatrician, or behavior specialist.

Will my stress urinary incontinence worsen over time?

Left untreated, the symptoms of your urinary incontinence are likely to worsen over time, since aging and gravity will continue to weaken your pelvic floor muscles. That is why it is so important to get a proper diagnosis, understand your treatment options, and choose a path toward healing as soon as possible.

Can stress urinary incontinence be cured?

Yes, women are often completely cured of their stress incontinence symptoms. In fact, the Agency of Healthcare Research and Policy reports that in 8 out of 10 women with urinary incontinence, symptoms can be improved.[10]

The likelihood of cure often depends on how early the condition is diagnosed, how soon after the symptoms start that treatment begins, how much time and attention you dedicate to your treatment (in the case of behavior modification or physical therapy, for instance), and how severe the loss of pelvic floor muscle function is.

Even if treatment does not completely cure your symptoms of stress incontinence, often it significantly reduces them so that they no longer interfere much with your day-to-day life. Your doctor or specialist will most likely follow a three-step procedure of screening, conservative treatment, and further evaluation.[11]

Step 1: Initial screening. To determine the cause of your urinary incontinence issues, the specialist will take a detailed medical history and ask you questions about your symptoms. Answer the questions as honestly and straightforwardly as you can. Be prepared to talk also about past gynecological or urological issues, prior surgeries, current medications, and any other medical conditions.

The physical examination will include a pelvic evaluation. This physical exam helps the physician determine the anatomy associated with your incontinence. During this evaluation, the specialist will determine whether any of your pelvic organs have prolapsed or fallen out of place, which may contribute to your urinary incontinence issues. The initial screening will probably also include the following tests:

- Urinalysis: This test helps rule out infection or blood in the urine as the cause of your urinary incontinence. You will be asked to provide a urine sample for testing. If the specialist suspects that you have a urinary tract infection, he or she will recommend a specific treatment plan to resolve the infection and send the sample for further testing. If blood is found in your urine, further testing may be needed to determine the cause.
- Post-void residual: As the name suggests, this test confirms whether you are fully emptying your bladder when you urinate. A catheter or ultrasound machine is used to measure the urine remaining in your bladder after urination. A normal post-void residual is less than 100 ml.

Step 2: Conservative treatment. At this point your physician will probably suggest nonsurgical treatment options, which we discuss later in this chapter.

Step 3: Further evaluation. If conservative treatment does not resolve your stress urinary leakage symptoms, your specialist may conduct further tests to understand more about your condition. These tests may include:

- Cystoscopy: A cytoscope is a thin, lighted viewing instrument that is inserted into the urethra and bladder. Your physician uses this instrument to examine the interior lining of the bladder and urethra for issues, other than weakened pelvic floor muscles, that may be affecting your continence.
- Urodynamics: This minimally invasive test focuses on your bladder's ability to fill and empty. It measures how much your bladder can hold, how much pressure builds inside your bladder as it stores urine, and how full it is when you feel the urge

to urinate. Urodynamic testing helps your doctor advise you about how well you might respond to certain treatments.

- Voiding diary: Your physician may ask you to keep a voiding diary as an essential part of your evaluation. This diary will allow you to communicate clearly with him or her about the status of your bladder, including how frequently you urinate during the day and at night, how much fluid you drink daily, and the volume of urine leakage you experience. The voiding diary will also educate you about your condition and may even amaze you. One woman was surprised, after keeping a voiding diary, that she needed to urinate 12 times a day, when 6 to 8 times daily is normal.

How do I talk to my doctor about stress urinary incontinence?

The key to having a successful doctor's appointment to address your urinary leakage issues is simple: preparation. Preparing for your appointment doesn't have to be complicated, but you should take the time to do so. Good preparation leads to good communication during the appointment. Your doctor gets all the information he or she needs to accurately evaluate your condition. You get answers to your questions and can explore your treatment options. You can prepare for your appointment in three easy steps.

Step 1: Observe your symptoms. If you have been dealing with symptoms of stress incontinence, this step may seem odd, since no doubt you are quite familiar with your symptoms. However, your doctor will probably ask you specific questions, so you will need to observe your symptoms closely for a few days and jot down notes. These notes will help your clearly describe your bladder symptoms during your appointment, even if you feel embarrassed discussing your situation. You may also want to write down any other health issues you experience, even if you think they are not related to your urinary incontinence. Finally, make a list of supplements and medications you take.

Step 2: Write your questions. The next step is to write a list of questions you have for your doctor. The list will come in handy during your appointment, reminding you to ask all your questions. For stress urinary incontinence, you may wish to ask your doctor about the following:

- Whether you have stress incontinence (it is important to have a clear diagnosis)
- Whether your symptoms can be improved or cured
- What kinds of tests you might need to assess your situation
- Whether lifestyle changes or diet modification might help
- What kinds of conservative treatments might improve your symptoms
- Whether your current medications could be aggravating your condition
- Whether other medications would help your condition
- Whether surgery is necessary
- Whether you should know about any other issues or factors related to this type of incontinence

Step 3: Gather your stuff and go. On the day of your appointment, gather up all your materials. You'll want to take your symptom list, your list of questions, as well as a notepad and pen so that you can write down important information during your appointment. If you were not able to list all the medications and supplements you are taking, simply gather all the bottles and pills into a bag and bring them with you to your appointment. If you have difficulty seeing or hearing, be sure to bring your glasses or hearing aids.

You may also want to ask a close friend or family member to accompany you to your appointment. Your companion can help you remember to ask all your questions and recall important information.

Your doctor may want to do a pelvic exam, especially if you have scheduled an appointment with a urologist or urogynecologist, so you may want to take special care with your personal hygiene before your appointment.

Then, having thoroughly prepared yourself, you are ready to fully explore the many available treatment options for solving your urine leakage issues. Lean on your buddy, your list, and your courage to get all the knowledge and help you need for your bladder symptoms.

What are my conservative treatment options for stress urinary incontinence?

Numerous conservative treatment options can be effective for improving or curing the symptoms of this type of urine leakage:

- At-home pelvic floor retraining
- Pelvic floor retraining guided by a specialist
- Medication
- Behavior and diet modifications plus weight management
- Acupuncture

At-home pelvic floor retraining.   If you are a do-it-yourself kind of woman, you may want to explore this treatment option. Chapter 7 of this book is entirely dedicated to helping you discover your level of pelvic floor fitness and teaching you exercises you can do daily to increase your pelvic floor tone. Improving your pelvic floor fitness can alleviate some or all of your symptoms, since stress urinary incontinence is caused by weakness in the pelvic floor muscles.

Pelvic floor muscle training is an effective treatment for stress incontinence, and some experts even recommend it as a first-line treatment for women with this condition.[12] Studies show that this kind of muscle retraining alone has an average cure rate of 73 percent. When combined with other conservative therapies, the average cure rate is 97 percent.[13]

Most doctors agree that pelvic floor muscle retraining is effective for treating this type of urine leakage but that the main problem with this approach is compliance. Women who follow a muscle-retraining program faithfully and correctly have a much higher success rate than women who don't follow the program correctly or consistently.[14] You should use this approach only if you know that you will be able to adhere faithfully to the recommended program.

For a complete description of the at-home pelvic floor retraining program, read chapter 7.

Pelvic floor retraining guided by a specialist. If you want or need more guidance in pelvic floor retraining, ask your primary physician for a referral to someone who specializes in this kind of therapy. Specialists include, among others, urologists, urogynecologists, nurses and nurse practitioners, physical therapists, geriatricians, and behavior specialists.

Some of these specialists are hands-on, meaning they will use various methods to evaluate the condition of your pelvic floor muscles and to teach you how to strengthen them. Some specialists may perform a pelvic exam to test the strength of your pelvic muscles, similar to the self-tests described in chapter 7 of this book.

In addition, they may use biofeedback units, mild electrical stimulation, or other tools to help you feel and see how to do a correct pelvic floor contraction. This kind of feedback is important because many women cannot locate the right pelvic floor muscles to contract without additional cues or electrical stimulation. According to a retrospective review by the American Urogynecologic Society, biofeedback cured 22 percent of women with urinary incontinence and significantly decreased symptoms for a further 43 percent of the women.[15]

Read more in chapter 8 about pelvic floor retraining guided by a specialist.

Medication. Medication is another conservative approach that offers many women relief from their stress incontinence symptoms. There are three main classes of medication that your doctor may prescribe to treat stress incontinence: tricyclics, antimuscarinics, and estrogen. Although these medications are not currently approved by the FDA to treat pure stress urinary incontinence, studies indicate that they do improve or even cure symptoms.[16]

- Tricyclic medication: This is an older class of drugs that has often been prescribed for depression. It alleviates symptoms of this type of incontinence by blocking the receptors that cause uninhibited bladder contractions. Examples include amitriptyline and imipramine.[17]

- Antimuscarinic medication: These drugs work by blocking the contractile receptors in the bladder and can also increase bladder capacity. Examples include darifenacin, fesoterodine, oxybutynin, solifenacin, and tolterodine. Most of these medications are available in an extended-release form, and oxybutynin is also available as a skin patch or gel.[18] These medications are FDA approved for urge urinary incontinence and mixed urinary incontinence, but they commonly improve stress urinary incontinence as well.
- Estrogen: Estrogen works primarily by thickening the lining of the urethra, which may help support the bladder and decrease symptoms of stress incontinence. It is available as a cream, tablets, or a time-release intravaginal ring. Many women with this kind of urinary incontinence report that estrogen relieves their urine leakage symptoms.[19]

Get complete details about the medications used to treat stress urinary incontinence in chapter 8, which describes additional conservative treatments for pelvic floor health.

Behavior and diet modifications plus weight management. You may have more control over your symptoms than you realize. Often women can decrease symptoms of stress incontinence by changing certain lifestyle habits. Most of these changes, recommended by the National Institutes of Health, are fairly simple:

- Bladder retraining: This involves learning to delay urination after you get the urge to go.[20]
- Stopping smoking: Smoking causes repeated and chronic coughing, which puts pressure on the bladder and pelvic region. Nicotine is also a bladder irritant. According to the National Association for Continence, when you stop smoking and coughing, chances are your symptoms will decrease.[21]
- Avoiding bladder-irritating foods: Certain foods can decrease the pH of your urine, making it more acidic. This can sometimes irritate the bladder and urethra, increasing the urge and frequency of urination. For instance, reducing your intake of

caffeinated drinks, alcohol, and acidic foods can make a big difference in your symptoms.

- Timing your fluid intake: To reduce symptoms of stress urinary incontinence, you can reduce fluid intake after 6 p.m. and drink most of the water you need for the day in the morning.
- Avoiding constipation: Straining to have a bowel movement puts pressure on the abdominal cavity, which can worsen your symptoms. Maintaining bowel regularity often decreases symptoms.
- Weight management: Every extra pound you carry puts additional pressure on your abdominal cavity, which can increase symptoms. Weight loss significantly decreases stress incontinence symptoms for many women who are overweight. In one study, sponsored by the National Institutes of Health, women who lost 8 percent of their body weight, or about 17 pounds, reduced their leakage incidents by almost half.[22]

Learn more about each of these behavior modification techniques, including how to retrain your bladder and maintain bowel regularity, in chapter 8.

Acupuncture. Though less popular than some of the conservative approaches for treating stress urinary incontinence, acupuncture can be an effective option for women who choose not to use medication and are unable to commit to behavior modification or physical therapy. Acupuncture provides a solid middle-of-the-road solution for these women.[23]

Read more in chapter 8 about how acupuncture is used to treat stress incontinence.

What are my surgical treatment options for stress urinary incontinence?

Advances in surgery offer new options for women with this type of urinary incontinence. These days, several minimally invasive surgical options can treat this condition. If conservative approaches do not resolve your symptoms to your satisfaction, you may want to consider surgery. Modern surgical techniques make surgeries to alleviate stress incontinence truly effective, and most are done on an outpatient basis.

The most common surgical repair for this form of urinary incontinence is the transobturator tape. With this minimally invasive surgery, a mesh tape is surgically placed around the urethra to support the bladder and urethra and to prevent leakage. Studies have shown that this tape procedure is about 80 percent effective for relieving stress incontinence symptoms.[24] Other surgical options include vaginal tape and the pubovaginal sling, with the sling having similar outcomes to the transobturator tape procedure.[25] Most gynecologists are also trained to perform older, well-established surgeries for stress incontinence that are more invasive, including the Burch procedure and the Marshall-Marchetti-Krantz procedure.

Don't let these names and surgical techniques scare you. Surgeries to treat this type of urine leakage can be quite painless for most women thanks to advances in modern medicine. At the same time, surgery is a more serious treatment option for stress incontinence, and if you are considering this approach, you will likely have questions about choosing the best surgeon, the possible side effects of surgery, aftercare procedures, pain management, and so forth.

The answers to these questions apply not only to surgical procedures that address stress urinary incontinence, but also to surgeries for other types of incontinence and pelvic organ prolapse. That's why we have placed detailed answers to these questions and more in a single easy-to-read chapter, chapter 9. If you are considering surgery for your urine leakage symptoms, or any other kind of pelvic floor repair, please read this chapter.

The more knowledge you have about your conditions, the better you can advocate for your health. Learn more about stress incontinence and urinary incontinence in general using the additional resources listed in the back of the book.

3

Overactive Bladder and Urge Urinary Incontinence

MY STORY:

Recovery from Overactive Bladder and Urge Urinary Incontinence

I knew I should have gone to the restroom before I left the grocery store. Now I can't get the keys in the door fast enough, and I'll probably have an accident. Hurry, open the door, push the dog out of the way, throw down the groceries, and pull down my pants. . . . Too late. Urine is running down my leg. Again.

I began having these episodes of suddenly needing to urinate about three years ago, after I went through menopause. It got so bad that I started looking for bathrooms everywhere I went—every mall, restaurant, theater, store, everywhere. It was driving me crazy. Then, when my doctor suggested I stop using estrogen because I had been on it for many years, the wetting accidents started. I'm not talking about a few drops. My whole bladder emptied once I got that urge. It was so embarrassing.

Then, over coffee with my daughter-in-law, we began discussing the maladies of aging, and she told me she'd had several urine leakage accidents, too. She was only 35. So she'd done some research online and learned that having accidents at any age is not normal. She suggested I talk to my primary care doctor at my next checkup. I was pretty embarrassed but I managed to raise the issue during the appointment, and he referred me to a specialist, a urologist.

The specialist asked me many strange questions. She wanted to know about my diet and how much coffee I drank. When I told her I drank two to three cups in the morning and one in the afternoon, she told me that coffee, tea, chocolate, and alcohol, as well as citrus fruits and spicy foods, could irritate my bladder and cause wetting accidents. She gave me a whole list of foods and drinks to avoid. She also asked me about constipation, and I admitted that I was chronically constipated. Apparently that can contribute to bladder problems, too. She recommended that I start fiber supplements to ease the problem.

After she did a pelvic exam, I learned that my pelvic organs were in good position, but that my pelvic floor muscles were not very strong. That was not a big surprise since I had delivered four babies vaginally— and they were pretty big babies.

She diagnosed me with urge urinary incontinence and gave me a list of conservative therapies and lifestyle changes to treat the condition. She said I needed to modify my diet, alleviate my constipation, and lose about five pounds. I was amazed that just five pounds could make such a difference in my condition. My urologist also wanted me to work with a pelvic floor physical therapist to strengthen my pelvic muscles.

I was so tired of the wetting accidents that I did exactly what the urologist recommended. I was thrilled when the frequency of the accidents decreased. The physical therapist gave me all types of exercises to do and used biofeedback to show me when I was engaging the correct muscles. She also used an electrical stimulation device to help with bladder relaxation. After working with her for six weeks, I started a home maintenance program. I was also pleased when the changes in my diet, including my fiber intake, resulted in a five-pound weight loss.

I did really well on this program for about two years, and then gradually I started to feel those strong urinary urges again. Sometimes I would start leaking urine before I could get to the restroom, especially at night, so I went back to the urologist.

After making sure that I had done everything she had recommended previously, she examined me again. Luckily all of my organs were still in the right places. My urologist asked me if I would like to try a medication to help suppress these urges. Although I was ready to try the medication, I had concerns about the side effects of constipation and dry mouth. My urologist assured me that increasing my water and fiber intake would prevent these problems.

The prescribed medication has made a big difference. I still have to watch my diet, fiber intake, and weight, but I can now go shopping, have lunch with my friends, and even sit through a whole movie. This medication, along with the lifestyle changes, has dramatically improved my quality of life. Now I feel like I'm 64 years young rather than an old lady.

Overactive Bladder and Urge Urinary Incontinence: The Surprising Flood

Most of us have experienced the effects of overactive bladder in our lifetime, including the strong urge to urinate or the need to urinate frequently. Some of us have also felt the symptoms of the most severe form of overactive bladder, called urge urinary incontinence. With urge incontinence, there is a sudden strong urge to urinate accompanied almost immediately by urinary leakage. Overactive bladder affects about 17 percent of women in the United States, with 9.6 percent of those women having urge incontinence.[1]

If you have overactive bladder, then you are familiar with the need to know the location of bathrooms wherever you go, since you need to urinate often and usually urgently. Even if you don't have this condition, you may have experienced urinary leakage from an episode of urge incontinence. This can occur in unusual circumstances, such as when you wait too long before you urinate because you are juggling too many things or don't have access to a restroom for a long time.

But if you experience chronic urge urinary incontinence, then you know firsthand that the situation is much more frequent and much worse. The urge to urinate comes on suddenly, followed by a strong bladder contraction resulting in leakage. Unfortunately, this form of urinary incontinence can be much more embarrassing than stress incontinence because the amount of urine leakage is frequently so large that the accident is difficult to hide. In fact, after leakage accidents, women with urge incontinence often have to change their clothing before they can move on with their day. Just imagine standing in line at the grocery store and leaking so much urine down your leg that it forms a puddle on the floor. If an incident like this has ever happened to you, then you know how incredibly embarrassing it can be.

You might feel the sudden urge to urinate when you hear water running in the kitchen sink or when you are trying to unlock the door with your arms full. Many women also leak when going from a sitting to a standing position, or when they wake up at night to go to the bathroom. There are numerous other triggers for urge incontinence, including tobacco use, immersion in cold water, and laughing hard.

Does that sound like you? According to recent studies, about 17 percent of women have overactive bladder, but only 13 to 51 percent of these women seek help for their condition.[2] Often, women with urge incontinence not only know the location of bathrooms everywhere they go, but they also carry several changes of clothes around with them in case they experience a leakage incident during the day.

Are you living in a shrunken world?

Fortunately, there are various treatments for overactive bladder and urge urinary incontinence, ranging from conservative approaches like medication therapy and behavior changes to a minimally invasive surgical procedure, all of which we discuss in this chapter. You should definitely seek treatment if you have either of these conditions. It is important to keeping your life rich and healthy.

If you are too embarrassed to get help, just consider the story of the frog in boiling water. Set a frog in boiling water, and it will immediately try to jump out. But set a frog in a pan of cold water, and it won't object; slowly turn up the heat, and it will not notice that it is being boiled until it is too late. Although this analogy is a bit extreme, we see women in our practices who live with extreme circumstances. Women, of course, are not frogs, but like the frog in this analogy, many live in a world that slowly changes until it reaches an extreme state. We call this state the "shrunken world."

If you don't think your world has shrunk because of urge incontinence or overactive bladder, ask yourself whether you avoid any of these activities because you fear urine leakage:

- Going to public places without nearby restrooms
- Sitting on a friend's couch
- Exercising at a gym or other public location
- Having sex
- Jumping on a trampoline with your children
- Joining friends for a girls' night out or "shop till you drop" marathon

If you avoid any or all of these situations because you fear urine leakage, then you are living in a shrinking world. The point is that these changes happen gradually, one step at a time, until you live an isolated existence. One day you may wake up and find that you have no social life. Not only that, you may even be afraid to visit the doctor for fear that you won't make it through the appointment without an accident.

If you do find yourself living in a shrunken world, don't worry, because it is never too late to seek help. If you are not yet living in a shrunken world but may be headed in that direction, then understand that it is never too *early* to seek help. The earlier you consult your doctor about your condition, the sooner you start on the journey to a cure.

Why you should get help now

There are so many reasons to get help for urinary incontinence the moment you experience the first symptom, whether it is a tiny trickle of urine or an uncontrollable flood.

First, chances are you don't want to be a woman living in an "incredible shrinking world." No one has a good time living in a limited world.

Second, plenty of research demonstrates that multiple conservative therapies are effective at improving or curing urge incontinence and overactive bladder symptoms. More important, the same research confirms that the sooner you get help, the more effective the treatment will be, because the effects of aging, gravity, and behavioral issues worsen with time.[3] If your condition is severe, minimally invasive surgical options are also available.

Third, knowledge is power. The more you know about your urinary incontinence, the better you can address your symptoms. Visiting your doctor, who will do several tests to determine the type of urinary incontinence you have, gives you the correct diagnosis. Once you have a diagnosis, you can learn the factors that contribute to your urine leakage. You may be surprised at how small changes in your lifestyle and behavior can positively affect and diminish your symptoms.

If you are ready to start the journey to recovery, and to learn more about urge incontinence and overactive bladder, then we strongly encourage you to read on. Throughout the rest of this chapter, we offer you the facts about these conditions, describe the tests that may be used in diagnosing your condition, and discuss multiple treatment options.

What You Need to Know about Overactive Bladder and Urge Urinary Incontinence

What exactly are overactive bladder and urge urinary incontinence?

Overactive bladder is a urinary condition caused by strong involuntary bladder contractions. With this bladder issue, you might experience any or all of these three symptoms: feelings of urgency to urinate, the need to urinate frequently, or urinary leakage. If you struggle with urinary leakage as a result of these involuntary bladder contractions, you have the most severe form of overactive bladder, urge urinary incontinence.

The International Continence Society recently defined overactive bladder as including symptoms of urinary frequency, nocturia (the frequent urge to urinate at night), and the sudden urge to urinate—sometimes singly and sometimes in combination.[4] Doctors who make this distinction also distinguish between overactive bladder with urge incontinence (called "overactive bladder wet") and overactive bladder without urge incontinence (called "overactive bladder dry").

You may or may not feel the urge to urinate when you leak urine due to urge incontinence. If you do have a strong urge to urinate, you may not be able to delay urination at all. When the process of urination works properly, the bladder muscles contract when enough fluid accumulates, usually about one cup (a healthy bladder can hold between one and a half and two cups of fluid). In healthy adults, the cerebral cortex in the brain controls when the bladder muscles contract, which allows a woman to "hold" her urine until she can reach a bathroom.

If you have urge urinary incontinence, the bladder muscles contract inappropriately and suddenly, often regardless of how much fluid is in the bladder. That is why women with this condition rarely have enough warning time to get to the restroom, resulting in urine leakage.

How common are overactive bladder and urge urinary incontinence?

As with all types of urinary incontinence, estimating the prevalence is difficult because many women who are coping with urine leakage do not seek help for various reasons. Embarrassment tops the list, followed by acceptance of urine leakage as a sign of aging.

Based on multiple studies and research, however, the most recent estimates indicate that overactive bladder affects about 17 percent of women in the United States. According to the National Overactive Bladder Evaluation (NOBLE) study, more than half of women with overactive bladder also have urge incontinence, which means they leak urine.[5] Urge urinary incontinence occurs more frequently in women than in men, especially in women age 44 or older. Both conditions tend to be more common in women age 45 or older, and there is a marked rise in urge incontinence in women age 64 or older. This differs from stress incontinence, which tends to be more common in women under 50. Urge incontinence has also been reported in 20 percent of young women athletes with eating disorders.[6]

(a)

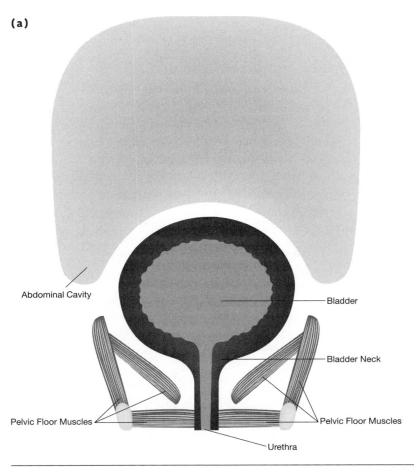

Abdominal Cavity

Bladder

Bladder Neck

Pelvic Floor Muscles

Pelvic Floor Muscles

Urethra

FIGURE 3.1. (a) Healthy bladder. (b) Overactive bladder/urge urinary incontinence bladder.

What causes overactive bladder and urge urinary incontinence?

Urge incontinence and overactive bladder symptoms tend to occur regardless of how much urine is in your bladder. Usually, in women with these conditions, the bladder is not as relaxed as it should be, and the bladder muscles contract involuntarily and frequently (see the comparison between a healthy bladder and an overactive bladder/

(b)

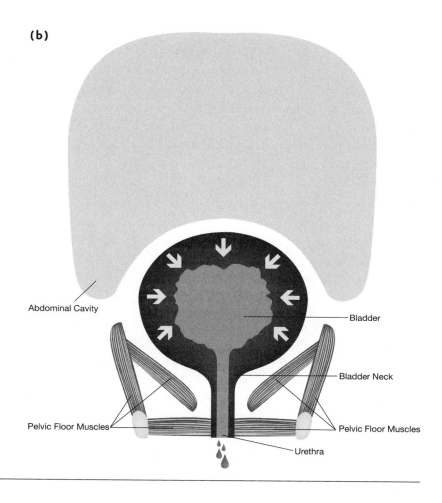

Abdominal Cavity

Bladder

Bladder Neck

Pelvic Floor Muscles

Pelvic Floor Muscles

Urethra

urge incontinence bladder in figures 3.1a and 3.1b). Doctors often describe a bladder in this condition as "physically unstable" and "spastic." This involuntary contraction of bladder muscles is commonly caused by abnormal nerve signals from the brain. For urinary leakage to occur, the pressure from the involuntary bladder contractions must exceed the closing pressure of the urethral sphincter (the seal that keeps urine in the bladder until you choose to urinate).

There are numerous possible causes of urge incontinence or overactive bladder, including bladder tumors, stones, or infections; hormone changes; problems with the bladder muscles or nerves; or neurological diseases (such as multiple sclerosis) or injuries (such as stroke or spinal cord injuries). Additional factors that may worsen this condition include certain foods and fluids, certain types of medications, anxiety or other troubled emotional states, excessive weight, and medical conditions such as hyperthyroidism or uncontrolled diabetes.[7] As the prevalence statistics demonstrate, aging is also a cause of these urinary conditions. Bladder cancer, inflammation, outlet obstruction (blockage), or, very rarely, urethral stricture (narrowing) may contribute to overactive bladder or urge incontinence.

How do I know if I have overactive bladder or urge urinary incontinence?

You know you have overactive bladder if you experience symptoms of urinary frequency (urinating at least eight times a day) or urgency (at least four times per month) and use at least one of these coping strategies: fluid restriction, immediately locating bathrooms in a new place, limiting travel, or defensive voiding (i.e., voiding before a movie so you won't have to get up during the movie to go to the bathroom).[8] Waking up at night to urinate is another symptom of an overactive bladder.

You know you have urge incontinence if you suddenly leak urine, often a large volume of it. Sometimes the involuntary urine loss is accompanied by a feeling of urge, but even if you feel the urge, chances are that the loss of urine will occur so quickly that you will not have a chance to find a bathroom.

What are the risk factors for overactive bladder and urge urinary incontinence?

The risk factors for these conditions include:

- Aging
- Obesity

- Smoking
- Being a woman
- Anxiety or similar emotional states
- Urinary tract infections
- Certain medications, like diuretics
- Low levels of estrogen, which can lead to bladder irritability and urgency
- Medical conditions like hyperthyroidism or uncontrolled diabetes
- Damage to nerves of the bladder, the nervous system, or the bladder muscles (caused by conditions like multiple sclerosis, Parkinson's disease, stroke, or injury)

Certain factors also tend to trigger urine leakage incidents:

- A sudden change in position or activity
- Touching or hearing running water
- Hard laughing
- Drinking small amounts of liquid
- Smoking tobacco
- Getting up at night to go to the bathroom
- Immersion in cold water
- Drinking certain liquids, such as coffee, tea, or carbonated beverages
- Eating certain foods, such as chocolate or those that are spicy, acidic, or tomato based

For a full list of foods and drinks that can irritate the bladder, and which you will want to avoid to prevent leakage accidents, consult chapter 8 on conservative therapies, specifically diet and lifestyle changes.

When should I contact a doctor about overactive bladder or urge urinary incontinence?

With all forms of urinary incontinence, you should seek help from your doctor if you have more than one episode. Studies show that the earlier urinary incontinence is treated, the more successful the treatment is, since aging, the effects of gravity over time, and certain lifestyle choices tend to worsen symptoms.[9] Yet despite the problem getting worse with time, most women experiencing urinary incontinence are too embarrassed to seek help. Women who do seek help often do not follow through with suggested conservative therapies.

In one study 65 percent of women coping with overactive bladder found the symptoms bothersome enough to adversely affect their lives. A surprising 60 percent of them sought help from a doctor, but 73 percent did not stay with the suggested medication (for reasons including cost, less-than-expected effectiveness, and significant side effects), and 46 percent were not likely to discuss the topic with their doctor again.[10] In general, only 13 to 51 percent of women with any kind of urinary incontinence seek help from the medical community. Women who experience frequent or severe leakage problems, or a significant drop in their quality of life, are more likely than average to seek help. But, and this is important, if the physician does not respond to the patient regarding her urinary incontinence problem, the patient is not likely to raise the issue again. Many interpret the doctor's silence to mean that there is no treatment. Perhaps for all these reasons, 70 percent of patients with overactive bladder have tried at least one non-medical coping mechanism before seeking help from a doctor.[11]

We strongly encourage you to be far more aggressive in seeking help than most women with these conditions are so that you can successfully resolve your urge incontinence or overactive bladder symptoms. Multiple treatment options have been shown to be effective for your condition, and by seeking help, you also avoid other related health issues, such as depression. Although about 30 percent of all women with urinary incontinence suffer from depression, that percentage doubles in women with urge incontinence—60 percent are depressed or have a history of depression. Getting treatment for urge incontinence or overactive bladder can also help you avoid related problems like falls and fractures (from rushing to get to the bathroom), skin infections, and a significant decrease in your quality of life, all of which are 2.8 times more likely to occur in women with either of these urinary conditions.[12]

If those facts are not enough to encourage you to call your doctor, consider this: seeking help can also lower your medical bills, since women with overactive bladder or urge urinary incontinence have medical costs similar to those of women being treated for osteoporosis or breast cancer.[13] If nothing else, the effect on your wallet of coping with urine leakage should motivate you to call your doctor.

Will my overactive bladder or urge urinary incontinence worsen over time?

Statistics indicate that both conditions will worsen over time, since they are more common among the older population of women. This is in part because of the hormonal changes associated with menopause. Left untreated, these urinary problems will worsen because the causes of the condition will continue. For instance, continuing to consume foods or drinks that irritate the bladder will cause the bladder muscles to continue to contract involuntarily. Plus, an irritated bladder can lead to more frequent urinary tract infections, which also worsen symptoms. Similarly, if a woman is experiencing urge incontinence because she is taking a diuretic medication for hypertension, continuing to take the same medication will ensure that her urine leakage symptoms stay the same or worsen over time. In short, without a proper diagnosis and treatment plan, urine leakage and other overactive bladder symptoms will continue regularly, with most symptoms getting worse over time.

Can overactive bladder or urge urinary incontinence be cured?

Many women can be cured of the symptoms of these conditions, and most experience symptom improvement with treatment even if they are not fully cured. In fact, the Agency for Healthcare Research and Quality (formerly known as the Agency for Health Care Policy and Research) reports that 8 out of 10 women with urinary incontinence can improve their symptoms.[14]

As with most types of urinary incontinence, most doctors agree that treatment of overactive bladder or urge incontinence begins with the least invasive approach that has the lowest risk of adverse events. This generally means conservative therapies such as behavior or life-style changes, including weight loss, diet change, smoking cessation, physical therapy, and acupuncture. Medication may also be needed. If conservative therapies and medication fail to improve or cure your symptoms, then your doctor may refer you to a surgical specialist to consider surgical procedures that address your condition.

Results are usually positive for conservative treatment. For instance, up to 70 percent of women report an improvement of urge incontinence symptoms from Kegels and other physical rehabilitation programs.[15] Most doctors report that a patient's success in resolving overactive bladder or urge incontinence symptoms depends on the severity of symptoms, the accuracy of the diagnosis, and the patient's perseverance with the prescribed treatment. With both of these urinary conditions, instant improvement is rare, but the overall prognosis is good in the long term.

How will my doctor diagnose whether I have overactive bladder or urge urinary incontinence?

For most women, talking to their doctor about urinary incontinence issues is embarrassing enough. Not knowing what procedures the doctor might use to diagnose a woman's condition may make her even more hesitant to raise the issue. That is why we review the basic procedures most doctors will use to evaluate urinary incontinence. Once you know how your doctor is likely to evaluate your condition, you can feel more comfortable getting help for your urinary incontinence.

Initial screening. First, it is important to know that your doctor will either diagnose your condition directly or refer you to a specialist, such as a urologist or urogynecologist. The tests your physician or the specialist will use to evaluate overactive bladder or urge urinary incontinence will be similar to those used to evaluate stress incontinence. In other words, he or she will do a detailed initial screening, which includes taking a full medical history and performing a thorough physical examination.

You can assist your doctor in this phase of evaluation by being prepared with the facts of your medical history. For instance, you want to be able to provide your doctor with details about the following:

- Your current urinary incontinence symptoms
- Any past and present medical conditions
- A list of medications you currently take
- Your voiding and leakage pattern over a week or so (also called a bladder, or voiding, diary)
- The amount of urine leakage per incident
- Recent surgeries and illnesses
- Causes of excess straining in the pelvic region, such as chronic coughing or constipation

In addition, your doctor will also perform a physical examination, including a pelvic exam, to discover if there is an anatomical cause for your urinary incontinence symptoms. Specifically, your doctor will evaluate the nerve function of your pelvis and check the position of your pelvic organs, including your bladder, rectum, uterus, and vagina. The physical exam will also reveal whether weakness in your pelvic floor muscles or other causes, such as fistulas (rare abnormal connections between the urinary tract and the vagina), may be causing your leakage issues.

Your doctor will also most likely do a urinalysis to determine whether an infection or blood in the urine is causing your symptoms. Another test you may likely undergo on this first visit is called a postvoid residual. This test helps your doctor evaluate whether any urine remains in your bladder after you have attempted to empty it, and measurement is usually conducted by catheterization or ultrasound. Any residual greater than 100 ml is considered abnormal.

If your doctor gathers enough information from this initial visit to make a diagnosis, he or she will most likely recommend conservative treatment. If your condition is severe, your physician may encourage you to consider surgical solutions as well.

Further testing. If you try conservative approaches (discussed later in this chapter) for your symptoms, such as pelvic floor rehabilitation or medication, but experience little or no relief from your symptoms, your doctor may perform further tests to gather more information about your condition. If you did not provide a voiding diary during your first visit, your doctor may ask you to keep one to provide a clearer picture of your leakage and voiding patterns.

In addition, the physician may perform a urodynamic test and a cystoscopy. A urodynamic test measures the volume of fluid your bladder can hold, the amount of pressure that builds inside your bladder as fluid levels rise, and the quantity of urine in your bladder when you feel the urge to urinate. Basically, urodynamic testing reproduces your symptoms in a monitored environment so that your doctor can learn more about the possible causes of your urine leakage.

For a cystoscopy, the physician inserts a very thin lighted scope into your urethra and up into the bladder. This allows your doctor to view the interior lining of your bladder and urethra, identifying any issues, other than weakened pelvic floor muscles, that may be causing your symptoms. Based on the information gathered from these two tests, your doctor can then recommend further treatment options for your symptoms.

How do I talk to my doctor about overactive bladder or urge incontinence?

It is important for you to be a strong health advocate for yourself, even when you're embarrassed, so that you don't find yourself living in the "incredible shrinking world" we discussed earlier.

In general, talking to your doctor about urinary incontinence of whatever type is the same. You need to first observe your symptoms, write down your questions, and then get all your needs met on the day of your appointment. Please review "How do I talk to my doctor about stress urinary incontinence?" in chapter 2 for the details of this three-step process.

It may help you to know the kinds of questions your doctor will probably ask. Most physicians in the United States will follow the guidelines issued by the Agency for Healthcare Research and Quality, a branch of the U.S. Department of Health and Human Services. According to these guidelines, physicians are encouraged to ask the following questions:

- Can you tell me about the problems you are having with your bladder?
- Can you tell me about the trouble you are having holding your urine?
- How often do you lose urine when you don't want to?
- When do you lose urine when you don't want to?
- What activities or situations are linked with leakage?
- Is it associated with laughing, coughing, or getting to the bathroom?
- How often do you wear a pad for protection?
- Do you use other protective devices to collect your urine?
- How long have you been having a problem with urine leakage?

What are my conservative treatment options for overactive bladder or urge urinary incontinence?

Although doctors tend to use medication to treat patients with these conditions, other treatments can also be successful. Your doctor will most likely recommend one or more of the following conservative treatments for your symptoms:

- At-home pelvic floor retraining
- Pelvic floor retraining guided by a specialist
- Medication
- Behavior and diet modifications plus weight loss
- Acupuncture
- Percutaneous tibial nerve stimulation

At-home pelvic floor retraining. This conservative therapy program has the benefit of offering you the privacy of doing pelvic floor exercises in your own home. Although pelvic floor retraining exercises, like Kegels, are most often used to treat stress incontinence, some women report relief from urge incontinence or overactive bladder symptoms when they use this method. The goal of this kind of conservative treatment is to strengthen the pelvic floor muscles to increase the function of the urethral sphincter. In addition, women with urge incontinence report that doing Kegel contractions when they feel the sudden urge to urinate often delays the urination and prevents leakage. Studies also show that pelvic floor retraining is more effective for treating urge incontinence symptoms when combined with bladder retraining.[16] We discuss this combination later in this chapter.

For women with symptoms of overactive bladder or urge incontinence, the goal of a thorough and effective at-home pelvic floor retraining program is to be able to do correct pelvic floor muscle contractions when the bladder contracts inappropriately. Doing these contractions can assist in calming the bladder. For a practical at-home pelvic floor retraining program you can start immediately, read chapter 7, which includes a progressive set of exercises that will benefit any woman.

Pelvic floor retraining guided by a specialist. If you are living with urge urinary incontinence, you can benefit from reading and using the pelvic floor retraining program detailed in chapter 7. However, many women have difficulty identifying and contracting the proper pelvic floor muscles necessary to maximize the effectiveness of these exercises. If you have tried Kegels and other similar pelvic floor retraining exercises with less than total success, it might be time to seek the help of a specialist for some hands-on help.

Pelvic floor retraining specialists can be physical therapists, urogynecologists, gynecologists, or other medical professionals. You may need to ask your primary doctor or urologist for a referral. A specialist can do manual physical therapy to assess the strength of your pelvic floor muscles and help you locate, by touch, the correct pelvic muscles to contract.

Additional tools can help specialists assess the contracting power of your pelvic floor muscles and help you locate and engage the proper muscles. These include biofeedback and electrical stimulation devices. Electrical stimulation involves sending a low-frequency electrical current to relax the bladder. The current is delivered by either vaginal or anal probe. Treatment sessions usually last about 20 minutes and are performed every one to four days. According to the National Institutes of Health, these are viable treatment therapies for women with symptoms of urge urinary incontinence or overactive bladder, and studies have shown that electrical stimulation therapy is effective at relieving symptoms.[17] The American Urogynecologic Society states that biofeedback is generally effective in improving urinary incontinence for 43 percent of women.[18]

Get more details in chapter 8 about working with a specialist for pelvic floor retraining.

Medication.   Four main classes of medication are used as conservative treatments for overactive bladder and urge incontinence: antimuscarinics, antispasmodics, tricyclics, and estrogen. Each of these medications has a different effect on the body, as well as different side effects. Your doctor may prescribe these medications singly or in combination.

- Antimuscarinic medication: This class of medications works by relaxing the muscles of the bladder to prevent the involuntary bladder contractions that cause these forms of urinary incontinence. There are several different medications in this class, and the six most commonly prescribed are oxybutynin, fesoterodine, tolterodine, trospium chloride, solifenacin, and darifenacin. Overall, studies indicate that no single antimuscarinic drug is more effective than any other for treating your symptoms, and you and your doctor may need to experiment with different types of this medication to find the one that works best for you. Between 16 and 23 percent of women with urge incontinence or overactive bladder experience complete continence with this type of medication.[19] This class of drug is generally well tolerated by most women, and some of the medications are available in multiple forms. Most are available in extended release and immediate release, and some are also available as transdermal patches. Oxybutynin is also available in a gel form, called Gelnique. The most common side effects of this class of drugs are dry mouth, constipation, and blurred vision.

- Antispasmodic medication: As with antimuscarinic medications, the goal of prescribing antispasmodic drugs for women with urge urinary incontinence is to calm the involuntary contraction of the bladder muscles. These drugs have been reported to increase bladder function and capacity. Two medications are more commonly prescribed for this condition than others in this class: hyoscyamine sulfate and flavoxate. Most antispasmodic drugs are available in both immediate release and extended-release formulations. Although this class of drug is prescribed for both overactive bladder and urge incontinence, studies are unclear as to its efficacy in alleviating symptoms. The side effects of this class of drugs are similar to those of antimuscarinic medications.
- Tricyclic medication: This class of drugs alleviates symptoms by relaxing the smooth bladder muscle to prevent the involuntary bladder contractions that cause urgency and leakage. Amitriptyline and imipramine are the most commonly prescribed. Studies reveal that these drugs are especially effective in alleviating nighttime incontinence, as well as in improving urge incontinence symptoms. The most common side effects of these drugs are sedation, dry mouth, dizziness, blurred vision, fatigue, and nausea.
- Estrogen: Topical estrogen is the most commonly prescribed for the treatment of symptoms. Recent studies show that estrogen is effective for treating symptoms of urge incontinence, although using it in combination with progestins may decrease its effectiveness.[20] Topical estrogen is available in a cream, pill, or long-acting ring.

Chapter 8 provides complete details about the different medications used to treat overactive bladder and urge urinary incontinence.

Behavior and diet modifications plus weight loss. Behavior and diet modifications have been shown to effectively improve symptoms of urge incontinence and overactive bladder. Changes in both lifestyle areas reduce the number of involuntary bladder contractions that result in involuntary leakage and excessively frequent urination.

More important, the guidelines for making these changes are easy to learn and use.

- Bladder retraining: This conservative approach works well if you are dealing with overactive bladder or urge incontinence symptoms because it retrains your bladder to contract when *you* choose to urinate, rather than contracting involuntarily or spasmodically. Bladder retraining basically consists of timed voiding, or urinating on a schedule. You start with a urination schedule to which you can comfortably adhere, such as every hour, and then gradually extend the period between bathroom visits. If you feel the urge to urinate between scheduled bathroom breaks, you do Kegel contractions to prevent leakage. You may also need to wear absorbent pads until your bladder becomes more accustomed to the voiding schedule.
- Avoiding bladder irritants: Anything that irritates the bladder can worsen symptoms because it increases the chances of involuntary bladder contractions. For instance, studies confirm that spicy or acidic foods irritate the bladder, as do caffeinated or carbonated drinks. Examples include food spiced with curry, chili peppers, or mustard, as well as citrus juices and coffee. Smoking can also increase urge incontinence leakage episodes due to bladder irritation.
- Timing and calculating fluid intake: The amount of fluid you drink, as well as when you drink fluids, can affect your symptoms. Most adults need between six and eight cups of fluids per day. This includes all the liquids you drink, not just water. Of course, you want to avoid caffeinated, carbonated, or citrus drinks, as mentioned above, and water is perhaps one of the healthiest fluids you can drink. If you are at either extreme of the weight scale, drink water in ounces equal to half your body weight (e.g., if you weigh 100 pounds, drink 50 ounces daily). If still thirsty, use sugar-free candies as needed to keep your mouth moist. Be sure to drink enough water because if your urine becomes too concentrated, it will irritate the bladder. Adequate water intake will also prevent constipation. Use an

over-the-counter mouth-moistening product if you experience dry mouth from your medications. If you are concerned about urine leakage at night, time your fluid intake so that you drink more fluid earlier in the day and stop drinking fluids after 6 p.m.

- Losing weight: While obesity or excess weight is more often associated with stress incontinence, anecdotal evidence suggests that weight loss can decrease urge incontinence or overactive bladder symptoms in obese or overweight women. Every extra pound above the pelvic floor increases the pressure on the bladder and can cause involuntary bladder contractions that lead to urine leakage accidents. According to the PRIDE study, which stands for Program to Reduce Incontinence by Diet and Exercise, losing even three pounds of weight can reduce leakage accidents by 25 percent.[21]

Get more details on all the behavior and lifestyle modifications you can make to improve your symptoms in chapter 8.

Acupuncture. Acupuncture is a useful conservative therapy to consider for women with overactive bladder or urge urinary incontinence whose symptoms are not sufficiently improved by medication, lifestyle changes, or pelvic floor retraining. Acupuncture is also useful when paired with other conservative treatments. This therapy seems to be effective because it affects the nervous system, and urge incontinence symptoms are caused by neural miscommunications between the brain and bladder.[22] Studies demonstrate that acupuncture does improve these types of symptoms, both according to medical evaluations and patient satisfaction reports.[23]

Chapter 8 offers more details about acupuncture as a treatment for urinary incontinence.

Percutaneous tibial nerve stimulation. This conservative treatment helps women with symptoms of overactive bladder or urge incontinence, including urinary leakage, urgency, and frequency. With this procedure, a fine needle is inserted just above the ankle, into the percutaneous tibial nerve (which helps control bladder function), and a mild electric current is delivered through the needle. Percutaneous tibial nerve stimulation produces a similar effect as sacral neuromodulation, a surgical treatment for overactive bladder and urge incontinence, but it is noninvasive and does not require surgery. This type of nerve stimulation usually requires three to four weekly visits to your urologist, with each appointment lasting 30 to 60 minutes. The treatment period spans 8 to 12 weeks. Patients who receive percutaneous tibial nerve stimulation experience up to a 20 percent reduction in urinary frequency, and more than a 35 percent reduction in the severity of symptoms.

Read the details about percutaneous tibial nerve stimulation in chapter 8.

What are my surgical treatment options for overactive bladder or urge urinary incontinence?

Research shows that the best surgical option for women with overactive bladder or urge incontinence who have not had success with conservative treatments is sacral neuromodulation, also called sacral nerve stimulation. This minimally invasive surgery implants a device that sends mild electrical pulses to nerves that control the bladder, pelvic organs, and pelvic floor muscles. The device is generally implanted in the buttock, under the skin. A thin lead wire is then anchored near the sacral nerve so that electrical pulses can stimulate the relevant pelvic nerves.

Studies reveal that this surgical solution is quite effective for women with overactive bladder, including urge incontinence. Sacral neuromodulation provides a cure for 31 percent of women who experience urinary urgency and frequency and improves these symptoms for a further 33 percent of women. This surgery provides a cure for up to 65 percent of women who have urge incontinence leakage, and a further 34 percent experience an improvement in this symptom.[24]

Learn more about sacral neuromodulation and other surgical procedures for urinary incontinence, pelvic organ prolapse, and decreased sexual satisfaction in chapter 9. See the additional resources listed at the back for more information about overactive bladder and urge urinary incontinence.

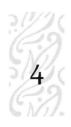

4

Mixed Urinary Incontinence

MY STORY:
Recovery from Mixed Urinary Incontinence

I was chatting with Resa over coffee one cold January morning, but I was holding back. I was reluctant to mention that I had an appointment with a specialist to talk about the urinary leakage problems I had been having for the last three years.

The problems had started after giving birth to my second child, my daughter. I leaked small amounts when I tried to go back to jogging to rid myself of the baby weight. But then after my second son was born, my third vaginal delivery, the problem worsened. Initially the leakage didn't happen often. I would be bathing the baby in the kitchen and suddenly get this terrible urge to urinate. At first I could control it, but eventually, since I couldn't leave the baby, the urine would just come. Gosh, I was only 35. I thought these problems only affected old people.

Finally, I took a deep breath and broached the subject. I told Resa about my appointment. To my surprise Resa had also seen a specialist for the same reasons. I was so relieved that I asked Resa what the doctor had done to help her. Resa said, "She told me that I had mixed urinary incontinence, and put me on this medicine to make the bladder relax and be a better container. She also sent me to a physical therapist to increase the strength of my pelvic muscles so I wouldn't leak when I exercised or sneezed."

I asked Resa what sort of medicine she was taking and what the side effects were. My friend said the medicine was an antimuscarinic and that the main side effects were dry mouth and constipation. She explained that to combat the dry mouth she sucked on sugarless gum or candy, and she had increased the fiber in her diet to help with the constipation. She had also been visiting the therapist once a week and was learning how to strengthen her pelvic floor muscles by following the therapist's instructions and doing the prescribed exercises regularly. The therapist had used biofeedback to help Resa track and understand her progress.

Wow. I had been sure I would need surgery to solve my leakage problems. What a relief to know there were other options, especially since I might want to expand my family even further. Resa admitted that she had waited four years to get help because she had been embarrassed, too, and thought incontinence was a problem of the elderly. We laughed together, and even though I felt a little wetness on my panty liner, I looked forward to the day when I would not.

Mixed Urinary Incontinence: The Best and Worst of Both Worlds

In the last two chapters we discussed two types of urinary incontinence: stress incontinence and overactive bladder, which includes urge incontinence, the most severe form of overactive bladder. With stress urinary incontinence, you leak urine anytime the intraabdominal pressure increases, such as when you cough, sneeze, or even step off a curb. With overactive bladder, you experience sudden and frequent urges to urinate. With the most extreme form of overactive bladder, urge incontinence, you not only experience sudden strong urges to urinate but also leak urine, sometimes a large volume.

What if you experience symptoms of both stress *and* urge incontinence? Then you are probably dealing with mixed urinary incontinence, which is a combination of the two. The reason we call mixed incontinence "the worst of both worlds" is that women with this condition typically report more severe and frequent symptoms than women with just stress or urge incontinence.[1] For instance, women with mixed urinary incontinence tend to have more leakage accidents, more frequent urination, and more episodes of urgency to urinate. In addition, women with mixed incontinence rate their quality of life as more severely affected by urinary incontinence than women with urge or stress incontinence alone.[2]

In other words, women with mixed urinary incontinence suffer the most of all women who have urinary incontinence. That means a lot of women are struggling, since about one-third of all women with urinary incontinence have mixed incontinence.[3] That's the bad news. Luckily, there is also good news for women with this form of incontinence.

The good news about mixed urinary incontinence

Although mixed incontinence affects quality of life more severely than other forms of incontinence, this also means that women with a mixed condition are more likely to seek help from a doctor or other medical professional. Women faced with this condition are less able to simply cope with their symptoms. They are less likely to live in the "shrinking world" we discussed in chapter 3. Studies show that the severity of a woman's urinary incontinence symptoms predicts the likelihood of her seeking help.[4]

What these facts mean for you is that your doctor or specialist sees more women with mixed incontinence than women with pure stress or urge incontinence.[5] In other words, your doctor is likely to be familiar with your condition and the available treatments. Your doctor will probably determine which form of urinary incontinence is worse, stress or urge, and treat the dominant type first. This approach often takes care of most mixed incontinence symptoms, because they are usually driven primarily by one type of incontinence.[6]

If you are among the women suffering from mixed urinary incontinence who have *not* sought professional medical help, now is the time to seek assistance. Because mixed incontinence symptoms are often more severe than those from stress or urge incontinence, the relief you will feel when these symptoms are alleviated will be greater.

You can get help now simply by reaching out to your doctor. At the same time, you can help yourself by learning more about mixed urinary incontinence. In the rest of this chapter, we cover basic facts about this condition, how your doctor will evaluate your condition, and the many treatment options available to you.

What You Need to Know about Mixed Urinary Incontinence

What exactly is mixed urinary incontinence?

Mixed urinary incontinence is a condition in which both stress and urge incontinence symptoms are present. With stress incontinence, you experience urine leakage when you cough, sneeze, exercise, lift heavy objects, or do any activity that increases pressure in the abdomen. With urge incontinence, you experience the sudden urge to urinate, such as when you hear the sound of water running, accompanied by an involuntary bladder contraction and urine leakage. If you are experiencing mixed incontinence, you can leak urine under any of these conditions.

Mixed urinary incontinence falls into two categories, depending on whether the stress or urge incontinence symptoms are more defined. When stress incontinence symptoms are stronger, the patient is said to have "stress predominant–mixed urinary incontinence." With urge urinary incontinence symptoms more defined, the patient is categorized as having "urge predominant–mixed urinary incontinence."[7] The International Continence Society defines mixed urinary incontinence as "the complaint of involuntary leakage associated with urgency and also with exertion, effort, sneezing or coughing."[8]

How common is mixed urinary incontinence?

About one-third of all women who have urinary incontinence are experiencing mixed incontinence. Since both stress and urge urinary incontinence become more common with age, mixed incontinence is also more likely to occur as you age.

What causes mixed urinary incontinence?

Because mixed incontinence is a combination of urge and stress incontinence, it is caused by the factors that cause both of these independent conditions. For instance, the stress part of mixed incontinence is caused by weakened pelvic floor muscles or prolapsed pelvic organs, which result in instability of the bladder or urethra, causing urinary leakage. Urge symptoms are caused by frequent and involuntary contractions of the bladder due to abnormal nerve signals from the brain. Leakage from these involuntary bladder contractions occurs when the pressure from the contraction is strong enough to push urine past the urethral seal. Learn more about the specific causes of stress and urge urinary incontinence in the previous two chapters about these conditions.

Some women who report themselves as having mixed urinary incontinence may not have both stress and urge incontinence. Studies show that when urodynamic testing was performed to determine whether women reporting mixed incontinence had both physical bladder or urethral instability (stress incontinence) and involuntary bladder contractions (urge incontinence), most of these women did not. The majority showed severe stress incontinence symptoms as a result of bladder or urethral instability, but no bladder overactivity.[9]

Research also shows that the more severe a woman's urinary incontinence symptoms, the more likely she is to report mixed symptoms. Many doctors now believe that many women reporting mixed symptoms actually have severe stress incontinence, and some women have severe urge incontinence. It is likely that when incontinence episodes are frequent and severe, and they occur over a long period, the episodes tend to blur, and women have difficulty remembering the details related to each episode. The distinctions between the types of symptoms become unclear. This could explain why treating the more dominant form of incontinence, which is usually stress incontinence, resolves mixed symptoms for many women.[10]

How do I know if I have mixed urinary incontinence?

You know you have mixed urinary incontinence if you experience both stress and urge incontinence symptoms. If your leakage symptoms are severe, it may help to keep a voiding diary to track them. If you have severe symptoms, it is possible to confuse stress and urge leakage episodes.

To keep a voiding diary, make a note each time you urinate or have a leakage accident. Note the time, the amount of urine voided or leaked, and whether leakage accidents were related to stress incontinence (such as when you sneeze) or urge incontinence (such as when you feel a sudden unexpected urge to urinate when you hear the sound of running water). If you are unsure about whether an episode is related to stress or urge, read chapters 2 and 3 for details on each condition.

After a week or two of keeping your voiding diary, examine it to determine whether you have both stress and urge leakage episodes. If you do, then you have mixed urinary incontinence. Your voiding diary will also be an important diagnostic tool for your doctor, who will determine whether your symptoms are stress or urge dominant.

What are the risk factors for mixed urinary incontinence?

Risk factors for mixed incontinence are the combined risk factors for urge and stress incontinence. Please read chapters 2 and 3 for detailed lists of risk factors for each of these conditions.

When should I contact a doctor about mixed urinary incontinence?

The pelvic floor conditions we describe change from chapter to chapter, but the advice remains the same: contact your doctor for help as soon as you notice symptoms, especially if you have more than one episode.

The sooner you get help the better you will feel. This is especially important if you have mixed urinary incontinence since, as we pointed out earlier, women with mixed incontinence tend to experience more severe symptoms than women who have just one type of incontinence. In addition, if you have mixed symptoms, chances are that coping with your condition costs you more than if you had only one urinary incontinence issue. If the average woman spends more than $1,000 per year on adult diapers and laundry bills to cope with urinary incontinence, you probably spend more to cope with your condition since mixed urine leakage episodes tend to be more frequent and severe.[11] Because of the severity of your symptoms, you are also likely to be more motivated to seek help than women with only stress or urge incontinence. In short, get help and get help now.

Will my mixed urinary incontinence worsen over time?

Yes. Both urge and stress symptom worsen over time if left untreated, so mixed symptoms will also become worse over time. Both stress and urge symptoms are more common among older women. This means that mixed urinary incontinence, which is a combination of both conditions, will become more severe as you age. In addition, without treatment, the core conditions that cause mixed incontinence remain unaddressed, so you can expect your symptoms to progressively affect your quality of life.

Can mixed urinary incontinence be cured?

Because mixed incontinence is a combination of stress and urge incontinence, and both of these conditions can be successfully cured with conservative or surgical approaches, mixed urinary incontinence can also be cured. Many women are cured, and others experience significant symptom improvement. Your doctor will assess your condition and focus on treating the dominant urinary incontinence condition, either stress or urge. Research shows that when the dominant condition is successfully treated, the majority of mixed symptoms are also resolved. In some women, though, the secondary condition will also have to be treated. For instance, if stress incontinence is the dominant condition, and you have surgery that cures your stress incontinence symptoms yet you still suffer from urgency, you may need to take medication to address your urge incontinence symptoms.[12] Once you discover whether your mixed incontinence is stress or urge dominant, please read the relevant chapter to get the details on cure rates.

How will my doctor diagnose whether I have mixed urinary incontinence?

Your doctor will diagnose your condition with the same methods used for diagnosing urge or stress incontinence. The first step is an initial screening, which includes taking a detailed medical history and performing a thorough medical examination (including a pelvic exam). You can assist your doctor during this initial screening by providing a voiding diary, especially since women with mixed incontinence can experience confusion about their symptoms. The initial screening will also involve a urinalysis and post-void residual.

If necessary, your doctor may follow up with urodynamic testing, which will clarify whether you have the anatomical weaknesses associated with both stress and urge incontinence. Patients with true mixed incontinence have a physically unstable bladder and urethra as well as sudden involuntary bladder contractions. Both anatomical weaknesses will become apparent with urodynamic testing. Cystoscopy is another test your doctor may perform to rule out other causes of your urinary incontinence, such as tumors or abnormalities in your bladder. Read chapters 2 and 3 for more details on the tests your doctor may use to diagnose your condition.

How do I talk to my doctor about mixed urinary incontinence?

Talking to your doctor about mixed incontinence is the same as talking to your doctor about urge or stress incontinence. It takes the same amount of courage, and you need to provide the same kinds of information. To find out how to prepare for your doctor's appointment, as well as which questions your doctor is likely to ask, review the sections on talking to your doctor in chapters 2 and 3.

What are my conservative treatment options for mixed urinary incontinence?

The best conservative treatment for your mixed urinary incontinence will depend on whether your stress or urge symptoms are predominant. Your doctor will likely discuss any or all of these options:

- At-home pelvic floor retraining
- Pelvic floor retraining guided by a specialist
- Medication
- Behavior and diet modifications plus weight loss
- Acupuncture

Once your doctor has determined whether urge or stress incontinence is dominant, you can learn about the success rates of each of these conservative approaches for your dominant urinary incontinence condition.

You can also learn more about specific conservative treatment options in chapters 7 and 8.

What are my surgical treatment options for mixed urinary incontinence?

If urge incontinence is the dominant aspect of your mixed condition, then sacral neuromodulation is the best surgical option for treating you. Read more about this surgical procedure in chapter 3. If stress incontinence is predominant, you have a wide range of surgical options, depending on the severity of your symptoms and the type of anatomical weakness. Read chapter 2 for more details. For the specifics and success rates of all surgical approaches, read chapter 9.

Learn more about mixed urinary incontinence by consulting the resources listed at the end of the book.

5

Pelvic Organ Prolapse

Recovery from Pelvic Organ Prolapse

I have always been physically active, and at age 52 I am very proud of my fitness. Until recently I played tennis, cycled, or power walked just about every week. But one day, after changing out of my workout clothes at the local recreation center, I felt a strange bulging sensation between my legs when I squatted down to tie my shoes. I also sensed some pressure in my lower back.

I didn't understand what was happening, so I rushed home and stripped off my pants and underwear. I grabbed a hand mirror and put it between my legs. What I saw was a small bulge pushing out of my vagina. I had no idea what I was seeing in the mirror. My first instinct was to ignore the whole incident and hope it would all simply go away.

Luckily, I thought better of the situation and instead phoned my friend Natalie. I remembered that Natalie had once confided in me that she was having some "female problems," although I could not remember the specifics. Regardless, I figured that I could safely discuss my problem with her, without embarrassment. When I told Natalie what had happened at the fitness center, she immediately invited me over for a chat.

Over a cup of hot tea, Natalie reminded me that she'd experienced

63

urinary incontinence, not the strange bulging sensation I felt. But she remembered reading about my symptoms in the booklet that her urogynecologist had given her to help her understand her urine leakage problem. She dug around in her file cabinet and triumphantly pulled out a tattered pamphlet titled *Female Pelvic Floor Disorders*.

We flipped through the booklet until we came to a section labeled "Pelvic Organ Prolapse," which perfectly described that bulging sensation I had felt. After we had both read the section, Natalie turned to me and said, "You have got to call my specialist. She is great, and she can help you. Here's her number on the back of the pamphlet." Being a proactive woman, Natalie immediately handed me the phone with an expectant look.

Hesitantly, I called Natalie's specialist and made an appointment for the following week. I was reassured when I arrived at my appointment and discovered that the doctor was every bit as friendly and knowledgeable as Natalie had described. After taking a thorough medical history and doing a physical exam, including a pelvic exam, the doctor told me that I had a cystocele, a form of pelvic organ prolapse in which my bladder was herniated and pressing into my vagina.

She felt that the prolapse was the result of my age plus having given birth vaginally to my two daughters. Because of the size of the cystocele, my good health, and my age, the specialist recommended a cystocele repair surgery. She reassured me that the surgery would be an outpatient procedure and that I could likely return home the same day. Oddly enough, she also congratulated me for coming in right away, since apparently most women struggle for quite a few years before seeking help.

I wanted to continue my physically active life, so after discussing the surgery further, I agreed. The cystocele repair surgery went as promised, and I went home the same day, although I did need to use a catheter for a few days. After a six-week recovery period, I slowly returned to my fitness routine. Today I am just as active as I was before my surgery, and I never felt that bulging sensation again. I am so grateful that I called Natalie right away when I discovered the problem instead of suffering with the condition for years.

Pelvic Organ Prolapse: The Name Says It All

Pelvic organ prolapse is commonly referred to as POP, which is apropos since many women with this condition feel as though a bulge has "popped out" of their vaginas. Some women with severe pelvic organ prolapse also feel as though they are sitting on a ball. If you feel as though something has bulged or popped out in your pelvic region, chances are you have some form of prolapse in your pelvic area.

But not everyone with a prolapsed pelvic organ feels the symptomatic bulge or low-back pressure. Studies show that 4 to 10 percent of all women have severe enough prolapse to experience noticeable symptoms,[1] but that between 43 and 76 percent of women show some degree of prolapse during regular gynecological examinations,[2] even if they don't know they have it. There are other symptoms of pelvic organ prolapse that you may or may not associate with a problem in your pelvic region. These include feeling very full in your lower belly, urinary incontinence, experiencing pain during sex, and constant constipation. We discuss a full list of possible symptoms in the "How do I know if I have pelvic organ prolapse?" section, later in this chapter.

What to do before your pelvic organ prolapse starts to bulge

Studies show that strengthening your pelvic floor muscles with exercises like Kegels can help delay or even prevent pelvic organ prolapse symptoms.[3] Put this fact together with how common it is to have some degree of prolapse without having noticeable or strong symptoms, and you can easily arrive at two conclusions:

1. You would be wise to ask your gynecologist or urologist to look for signs of prolapse during annual checkups.
2. There is no better time than the present to start doing pelvic floor exercises to delay or prevent symptoms. If you already

have a pelvic floor exercise routine, you should definitely stick with it.

We stress in this book that knowledge is power. The more knowledge you have about your own body, the better you can act as your own health advocate. Another piece of knowledge you may want to add to your arsenal is whether your family has any history of hernias or pelvic organ prolapse. Scientists now understand that this kind of prolapse often occurs more frequently in women with a family history of hernias. In fact, women from families with a genetic predisposition for hernias are 1.4 times as likely to experience pelvic organ prolapse.[4] According to Dr. Mary McLennan, director of the urogynecology division of the Saint Louis University School of Medicine, "If your father has had a hernia and your mother has prolapse, you already have a risk of prolapse and should look at changing the things you can control to reduce your risk."[5]

Luckily, you can take many actions on your own to reduce your risk of prolapse or to decrease symptoms, including conservative lifestyle changes such as diet modifications, pelvic floor exercise programs, career choices that don't involve heavy lifting, weight control, smoking cessation, and more. There are also numerous surgical procedures that can successfully reverse the effects of pelvic organ prolapse. Next, we explore what you need to know about this condition to prevent or treat it.

What You Need to Know about Pelvic Organ Prolapse

What exactly is pelvic organ prolapse?

Pelvic organ prolapse is a condition in which one or more pelvic organs sags downward, sometimes noticeably and sometimes not. Different kinds of prolapse have different names, depending on which pelvic organs are prolapsed. Types of pelvic organ prolapse include prolapse of the bladder (cystocele), the rectum or large bowel (rectocele), the small intestine or small bowel (enterocele), and the uterus (procidentia). The suffix -cele comes from the Latin word for "hernia."

"Cyst" refers to the bladder; "rect" refers to the rectum; and "entero" refers to the small bowel.

How common is pelvic organ prolapse?

Between 4 and 10 percent of women will have prolapse with noticeable symptoms, and an estimated 7 percent of women will have surgery for prolapse by the age of 80.[6] About 3 to 6 percent of women have severe prolapse symptoms, meaning that organs have prolapsed below the vaginal opening, and these women will most likely feel as if they are sitting on a ball and may see an actual bulge outside their vagina.[7] But, as mentioned previously, between 43 and 76 percent of women who have pelvic organ prolapse don't experience noticeable symptoms. This condition is more prevalent in women older than 50.[8]

What causes pelvic organ prolapse?

Pelvic organ prolapse occurs when the tissues supporting the affected pelvic organ become weakened, causing a herniation. For instance, with a cystocele, the ligaments and muscles supporting the bladder wall are weakened and they separate, allowing the bladder to bulge down into the vagina (compare the normal pelvic anatomy to the pelvic anatomy with a cystocele shown in figures 5.1a and 5.1b). Similarly, with a rectocele, the rectal wall prolapses and presses against the back wall of the vagina (compare the normal pelvic anatomy to the pelvic anatomy with a rectocele shown in figures 5.2a and 5.2b). The small intestine prolapses into the upper wall of the vagina with an enterocele. In a procidentia, the uterus prolapses down into the vagina.

In all types of prolapse, gravity and giving birth are the most likely causes. In other words, the downward force of gravity over time, as we age,[9] as well as the effects of pregnancy and childbirth, particularly vaginal delivery,[10] can easily cause pelvic organs to prolapse.[11] However, there is no scientific evidence that elective cesarean sections decrease the risk of developing a prolapse.[12]

(a)

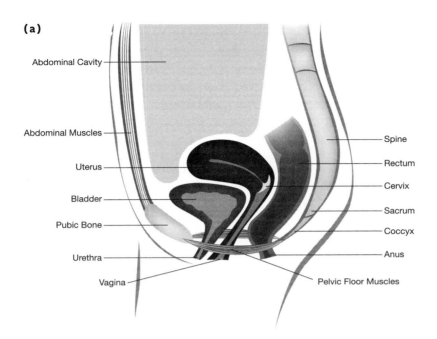

Abdominal Cavity

Abdominal Muscles

Uterus

Bladder

Pubic Bone

Urethra

Vagina

Spine

Rectum

Cervix

Sacrum

Coccyx

Anus

Pelvic Floor Muscles

(b)

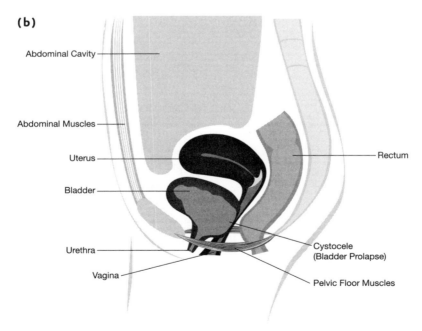

Abdominal Cavity

Abdominal Muscles

Uterus

Bladder

Urethra

Vagina

Rectum

Cystocele
(Bladder Prolapse)

Pelvic Floor Muscles

FIGURE 5.1. (a) Healthy pelvic anatomy. (b) Pelvic anatomy with a cystocele.

(a)

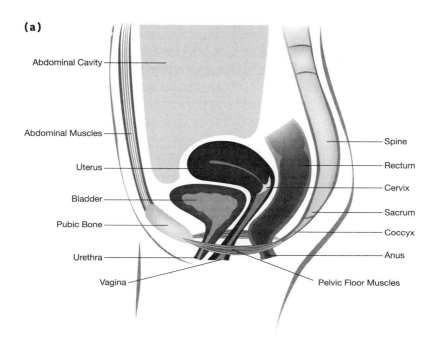

Abdominal Cavity

Abdominal Muscles

Uterus

Bladder

Pubic Bone

Urethra

Vagina

Spine

Rectum

Cervix

Sacrum

Coccyx

Anus

Pelvic Floor Muscles

(b)

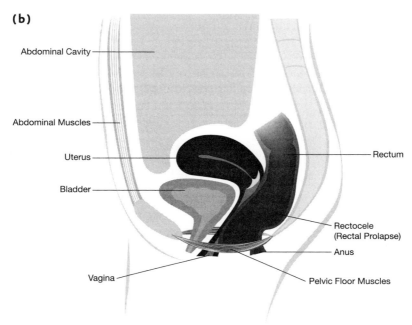

Abdominal Cavity

Abdominal Muscles

Uterus

Bladder

Vagina

Rectum

Rectocele
(Rectal Prolapse)

Anus

Pelvic Floor Muscles

FIGURE 5.2. (a) Healthy pelvic anatomy. (b) Pelvic anatomy with a rectocele.

How do I know if I have pelvic organ prolapse?

Since many women with prolapse do not have obvious symptoms, the best way to ascertain whether you have one is to have a thorough pelvic examination, usually done by a gynecologist, urologist, or other specialist. Symptoms of pelvic organ prolapse include:

- Experiencing pressure from pelvic organs pressing against the vaginal wall
- Feeling as if you are sitting on a ball
- Seeing a bulge pushing out of your vagina
- Feeling as if something is "falling out" of your vagina
- Experiencing urinary incontinence or frequency
- Having difficulty urinating (sometimes made easier by pressing on your abdomen)
- Being constipated (sometimes made easier by pressing your fingers in your vagina)
- Feeling a pull or stretch in your lower back or groin area
- Experiencing pain during sex

What are the risk factors for pelvic organ prolapse?

There are multiple risk factors for pelvic organ prolapse:

- Aging and menopause
- Vaginal birth, especially instrument-assisted delivery
- Pregnancy
- Prior pelvic surgery, such as a hysterectomy
- Genetic predisposition
- Obesity
- Constant straining, such as from chronic coughing or constipation
- Pelvic organ tumors
- Connective tissue disorders
- Smoking

- Diabetes[13]
- Long-term steroid use[14]
- Prior radiation for cervical cancer[15]

When should I contact a doctor about pelvic organ prolapse?

As with urinary incontinence, you should contact your doctor the first time you experience a symptom of prolapse. In addition, since you can have a prolapse without noticing any symptoms, you should have an annual pelvic exam. This lets you know whether you have any prolapsed pelvic organs. Since conservative measures, such as a pelvic floor muscle exercise program, can delay or even prevent prolapse, you want to find out if you have pelvic organ prolapse as soon as possible.[16]

Will my pelvic organ prolapse worsen over time?

Given that pelvic organ prolapse is more common in older menopausal women and that the effects of gravity only increase over time, an untreated prolapse is likely to worsen. There is no reason to delay treatment for pelvic organ prolapse. Conservative therapies like pelvic floor retraining or the use of a vaginal pessary can stabilize or even improve symptoms. For severe prolapse, surgical procedures have a strong rate of success (see chapter 9 for success rates of specific procedures).

How will my doctor diagnose whether I have pelvic organ prolapse?

Since genetics and family medical history play such an important role in prolapse, your doctor will first review your and your family's medical history. This history will include any other pelvic organ issues you may be experiencing, such as urinary incontinence or decreased sexual sensation. Your doctor will also note medications you take and any other health issues, such as recent illnesses or surgeries, or causes of excess straining in the pelvic region (such as obesity, chronic cough due to smoking, or chronic constipation).

After reviewing the medical history, your doctor will perform a physical evaluation, including a pelvic exam. During the pelvic exam your doctor will determine the strength of your pelvic floor muscles, whether any pelvic organs have prolapsed, and whether your bladder and urethra are stable. Additional tests may also include:[17]

- Urodynamic testing (measures your bladder's ability to store and empty urine)
- Magnetic resonance imaging, or MRI (creates a 3-D image of your pelvis), although a physical exam usually suffices since MRIs can be costly
- Cystoscopy (gives your doctor an inside view of your urethra and bladder)
- Ultrasound (assists your doctor in visualizing your kidneys, bladder, and other pelvic organs)

How do I talk to my doctor about pelvic organ prolapse?

Once you make an appointment with a specialist who can help you diagnose whether you have any prolapsed pelvic organs, it may help you to know ahead of time the questions your doctor will probably ask. You can jot down the answers ahead of time so that you make the most of your appointment. According to the Mayo Clinic, your doctor will probably ask some of the following questions:[18]

- What symptoms are you experiencing?
- When did you first notice these symptoms?
- Have your symptoms gotten worse over time?
- Do your symptoms include pain? If yes, how severe is the pain?
- Does anything in particular trigger your symptoms, such as coughing or heavy lifting?
- Do your signs and symptoms include urine leakage (urinary incontinence)?
- Have you had a chronic or severe cough?

- Does your work or do your daily activities involve heavy lifting?
- Do you strain during bowel movements?
- Are you currently being treated or have you recently been treated for any other medical conditions?
- What medications are you taking, including over-the-counter and prescription drugs as well as vitamins and supplements?
- Do any of your first-degree relatives—such as a parent or sibling—have a history of any organ prolapse or other pelvic problems?
- How many children have you delivered? Were your deliveries vaginal or cesarean?
- Do you plan to have children in the future?
- Do you have any other concerns?

In addition, you may also want to prepare your own list of questions for your doctor:

- Which type or types of pelvic organ prolapse do I have?
- What are my treatment choices given the severity of my symptoms, my family planning needs, and my surgical risks?
- What conservative treatment options are available to me, and what are the chances of these treatments relieving my symptoms?
- If I need surgery, what options are available? What are my chances of success? What are the chances that my prolapse will recur?
- Are there any activities that I cannot do during or after treatment?

What are my conservative treatment options for pelvic organ prolapse?

Multiple conservative treatment options are appropriate for women who have mild symptoms, wish to have more children, or are poor surgical candidates. In addition to monitoring and observation, these conservative measures include:

- At-home pelvic floor retraining
- Pelvic floor retraining guided by a specialist
- Behavior and diet modifications plus weight loss
- Vaginal pessary

At-home pelvic floor retraining. Pelvic floor retraining is one of the first-line conservative treatments for pelvic organ prolapse. Studies show that this kind of muscle retraining can reduce the severity of prolapse symptoms[19] and even delay the onset of pelvic organ prolapse.[20] Pelvic muscle retraining also improves pelvic muscle function, which has been demonstrated to help women with various urinary and pelvic symptoms.[21]

For a practical, easy-to-understand pelvic floor retraining program that you can start doing right away, see chapter 7.

Pelvic floor retraining guided by a specialist. Up to 50 percent of women cannot locate the correct muscles to do a pelvic floor muscle contraction based on written directions alone.[22] If you are among these women, or if you are just not sure whether you are doing these kinds of exercises correctly, don't be afraid to ask for help. You can ask your doctor for a referral to a physical therapist or other medical professional who specializes in pelvic floor retraining.

These specialists have specifically designed tools that can help you locate and engage the right muscles, including machines for mild electrical stimulation and biofeedback devices that alert you when you are using the correct muscles. These professionals also gently use their hands to help you feel and locate the muscles you need to engage.

Read chapter 8 for more information about pelvic floor retraining guided by a specialist.

Behavior and diet modifications plus weight loss. If you have a prolapsed pelvic organ, behavior modifications that can ease your symptoms include avoiding lifting heavy objects and not doing exercises that worsen your symptoms. If you smoke, or have other habits that cause you to chronically cough, stopping these habits can also help.

In terms of diet, eating extra fiber can help relieve constipation and prevent abdominal straining. If you have trouble urinating, then avoid foods (like citrus fruits), drinks (like caffeinated or carbonated beverages), and medications (like diuretics) that increase the urge and frequency of urination.

Finally, participating in mild exercise that does not worsen your prolapse and adjusting your diet so that you reach a healthy weight can help reduce pelvic organ prolapse symptoms. Every pound above your pelvic floor increases pressure on your prolapsed organs, so weight loss is always a positive conservative treatment.

Vaginal pessary. Your doctor can fit you with a vaginal pessary, a removable device that supports the sagging pelvic structures and relieves the pressure on your bladder and bowels. Pessaries come in various types and shapes, including rings, doughnuts, and cubes. With a supportive type of pessary, you can relieve pelvic organ prolapse symptoms and still engage in sexual activity.[23] Another advantage of a vaginal pessary is that it helps with all types of pelvic organ prolapse. The disadvantage is that it often requires one to three office visits to achieve a good fit and to find the right kind of pessary for your type of prolapse and the shape of your vagina. When fitting you for a pessary, your doctor needs to consider your prolapse symptoms, level of sexual activity, and your ability to insert and remove the pessary without assistance. Some pessaries cannot be removed except with the help of a doctor.[24]

From 70 to 90 percent of women report that their symptoms are resolved when using a well-fitting pessary.[25] An additional 40 to 60 percent of women with pelvic organ prolapse note an improvement in sexual activity.[26] Pessaries seem to be an effective method for alleviating prolapse symptoms, since at least half of all women who have well-fitting pessaries continue to use them for more than one year.[27]

What are my surgical treatment options for pelvic organ prolapse?

If your prolapse symptoms are severe enough, your doctor may recommend surgery. If you and your doctor decide on surgery, the surgeon will individualize the procedure for you, tailored for your type or types of prolapse. There are four main surgical repair procedures based on the type of pelvic organ prolapse:

1. Cystocele repair
2. Rectocele repair
3. Enterocele repair
4. Hysterectomy

If you are experiencing more than one type of prolapse, the surgeon will probably perform multiple pelvic organ prolapse procedures in the same surgery. The goal of the first three procedures is to restore the prolapsed organ to its original position; a hysterectomy entails the complete removal of the prolapsed uterus. Hysterectomies are usually performed by qualified gynecologists, but in certain circumstances, a urologist with special gynecological training can also perform this procedure. A hysterectomy may be performed in conjunction with the other prolapse surgeries. All of these surgeries are moderately invasive. Some are performed as outpatient procedures, and others require a short hospital stay.

Depending on the strength of your pelvic tissues, your surgeon may elect to repair the herniated tissue without the aid of mesh patches or donor tissue. If your surgery requires a mesh patch or artificial sling material, there is a small risk of mesh erosion or overtightening of the sling. With donor tissue, the associated risks are rejection or failure of the donor tissue. All pelvic organ prolapse surgeries have about the same types and amount of risk. All are performed under either general anesthesia or sedation with spinal (regional) sedation. Although on average 13 percent of women who have prolapse surgery will require a repeat procedure within five years, the overall success rates for prolapse surgeries are high (83 percent and above).[28]

Learn more about all pelvic organ prolapse surgical procedures in chapter 9. See the resources listed at the end of the book for additional information about pelvic organ prolapse.

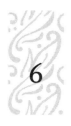

6

Decreased Sexual Sensation

MY STORY

Recovery from Decreased Sexual Sensation

Sex with my husband was great . . . and then it wasn't so great. Then it became a marital problem. After I had my kids, I just wasn't interested in sex. In fact, I avoided it altogether. I even got undressed in the closet so my husband wouldn't see me naked and get aroused. Then I figured maybe that happened to lots of moms, but when I checked with my friends, I discovered that this situation wasn't as common as I had thought. So after 10 years, when my lack of interest in sex had blossomed into a big issue in my marriage, I finally decided to get help from my gynecologist.

During the pelvic exam, she tested the strength of my pelvic floor. What she told me afterward made so much sense. I learned that a woman's state of sexual arousal and fulfillment can be affected by several factors, including the level of physical sensation. Women don't have much sensation in the vagina. Instead, they experience enjoyable sexual sensations when the pelvic floor muscles contract and expand against a man's penis. The stronger a woman's pelvic floor muscles, the more pleasurable the sensation she is likely to feel during sex. Apparently my pelvic floor muscles were weakened and stretched from having babies, which meant I didn't experience much sexual sensation. This also explained my lack of interest in sex.

My gynecologist referred me to a physical therapist, who evaluated my condition and taught me to strengthen my pelvic floor muscles by doing various Kegel exercises. After completing the physical therapy program, my therapist suggested that I continue to tone these muscles throughout my life. I enrolled in a Pilates course so that I could learn to engage my pelvic floor muscles during my regular exercise program.

The results have been incredible. Not only can I do a killer Kegel contraction with my pelvic floor muscles, but I also have sensation during sexual intercourse, much like I did before having children. My husband and I are excited about the results, and the time and effort I put into toning my pelvic floor has truly paid off. I strongly recommend that any woman suffering from loss of sexual sensation discuss this with her physician and ask for help.

Decreased Sexual Sensation: You Can Do Something about It

Is sex not as pleasurable as it used to be? Has sex never been as good as it could be? If so, then you may be experiencing decreased sexual sensation as a result of pelvic floor weakness. Many women are not even aware of their level of pelvic fitness, but all women can be affected by poor pelvic floor tone, which can lead to decreased sexual sensation as well as other symptoms:

- Unsatisfactory sexual response
- Low sex drive
- Pain during intercourse
- Urinary incontinence during sex

If you experience any of these symptoms, you may feel better knowing that other women feel the same way. Studies show just how many women are truly unsatisfied in the bedroom, often because of decreased sexual sensation and its accompanying symptoms.

- Orgasm difficulties affect 24 percent of women.[1]
- About 10 percent of women have never experienced an orgasm.[2]
- Between 33 and 50 percent of women are unhappy with how often they achieve orgasm.[3]
- More than 40 percent of women are dissatisfied with their sex lives.[4]

Sadly, the same types of research that produced the statistics above also show that women with unsatisfactory sex lives often settle for mediocre sex rather than seeking help. You should not settle when good sex can be had with a little extra effort.

Good sex and pelvic floor strength

Although there can be multiple reasons for unsatisfactory sex, many women—especially postpartum or older women—are less than satisfied with their sex lives for a single reason: decreased sexual sensation. Decreased sexual sensation is an indicator of a weak pelvic floor, which can definitely lead to unhappiness in the bedroom.

Most women, even those who are otherwise physically fit, don't spend much time thinking about their pelvic floor muscles. This is not surprising since these muscles are internal and not available for visual inspection. Thus the old adage "out of sight, out of mind" tends to apply to these muscles. Yet the pelvic floor muscles are vital to satisfactory sex. Here's why:

- Pelvic floor muscles are directly responsible for how much sensation a woman feels during intercourse.[5]
- Toned pelvic floor muscles are tighter and thicker.[6]
- Tighter, thicker pelvic floor muscles experience more stretch from an erect penis.[7]
- Firm muscles have more nerve endings, which means more pleasurable sensation from the stretch.[8]
- Toned pelvic muscles also have more circulation, which helps to engorge the clitoris and increases sexual sensation still more.[9]

You can see how toned, tight, and strong pelvic floor muscles are important to good sex. Luckily, even if you don't often pay attention to these muscles, there are many doctors, therapists, and researchers who do. From the clinical experience of these professionals, we now know that women can recover from decreased sexual sensation, often with a simple exercise program designed to strengthen the pelvic floor muscles in addition to other conservative measures. If the simplicity of this approach is not enough to get you started with a pelvic floor muscle exercise program, which we cover in full detail in chapter 7, then the next section on why good sex is good for you definitely will.

Good sex is good for you

If you have had satisfactory sexual experiences, then you know that good sex makes you feel great. But there is more to good sex than it being its own reward. Researchers have now demonstrated that good sex is good for you in many parts of your life. For instance, you may not know that

- Women with higher reported levels of sexual satisfaction also report a higher sense of purpose in life.[10]
- Sexually satisfied women are happier.[11]
- Women who explore ways to have a better sex life, with expectations for improvement, can experience better sexual well-being.[12]

These three inspiring findings should encourage you to pay attention to your pelvic floor muscles and learn more about how you can exercise and support these muscles for better experiences in the bedroom—and in life. The rest of this chapter tells you everything you need to know about decreased sexual sensation and how to alleviate this condition and its accompanying symptoms. Read on to learn more about the causes of this condition as well as the numerous treatment options.

What You Need to Know about Decreased Sexual Sensation

What is decreased sexual sensation?

Decreased sexual sensation is a condition in which women experience less sensation or less satisfactory sensation during sex. An affected woman may experience little to nothing in her genital organs, such as her clitoris and vagina. As a result, she may have a low libido, meaning she has little or no interest in sex, and may have difficulty achieving orgasm during sex.

How common is decreased sexual sensation?

As with other pelvic floor conditions, it's difficult to pin down the exact number of women affected by decreased sexual sensation since many women don't discuss the issue with their health care practitioners. But some studies give us an idea of how common this condition is:

- According to a 2005 study published in the *American Journal of Obstetrics and Gynecology*, sexual dysfunction affects 48 percent of women, and these same women had decreased sexual sensation specifically in their clitoris, which increased the chances of sexual dysfunction.[13] Other studies have found that more than 40 percent of women report sexual dissatisfaction.[14]
- The 2010 *National Survey of Sexual Health and Behavior* illustrates a large "orgasm gap," with 85 percent of men reporting that their partners experienced orgasm at their most recent sexual event, while only 64 percent of women report having an orgasm at their most recent sexual event.[15]

What causes decreased sexual sensation?

A common cause of decreased sexual sensation is having pelvic floor muscles that are either weak or damaged. These muscles are directly involved in how much sensation a woman experiences during sex. The vagina alone has relatively few sensory nerves, so most of the sensation during sex comes from the muscles that surround and support the vagina.[16] Visualize these muscles as a figure 8 that wrap around the vaginal and anal openings as well as the clitoris. This group of muscles is called the pubococcygeus, sometimes referred to as the "love muscle." Most women experience pleasure during penetration from the tension created by the pelvic floor muscles as the penis moves against them. One landmark study demonstrated that a woman's ability to orgasm was significantly related to the strength, or "squeeze pressure," of her pubococcygeus.[17]

Women with weak pelvic floor muscles usually don't know that they need to exercise these muscles, just as they would any other muscles in their bodies. As women age, they are at greater risk for weakened pelvic muscles, since these muscles will begin to lose tone and sag. In addition, as women reach menopause, their bodies produce less estrogen, which causes the vaginal tissues to become thinner and weaker. The result of all these changes is often decreased sexual sensation and a reduced ability to experience orgasm.[18]

Younger women can also experience decreased sexual sensation because of weak or damaged pelvic floor muscles. These muscles can be damaged by sports or exercises that involve a lot of jarring or jumping—such as cheerleading or gymnastics—or that put pressure on the genital area, such as long-distance bicycling. Studies show that more women cyclists (who consistently rode 10 miles per week) experienced decreased sexual sensation compared with women runners.[19] Women can also damage these pelvic muscles during childbirth, which can stretch and tear the muscles. This has a direct impact on a woman's sexual sensation because nerves within the pelvic muscles can stretch only 15 percent before damage occurs.[20]

How do I know if I have decreased sexual sensation?

Most women notice decreased sexual sensation after a life change, such as childbirth or a sports injury. Some women notice this condition as they approach or enter menopause.

You know you have decreased sexual sensation if you experience less sensation or almost no sensation during sex. Some women with decreased sexual sensation report that sex isn't uncomfortable, but they simply don't have much feeling in their sexual organs. Although some women notice a drop in the level of their sexual sensation, other women affected by decreased sexual sensation have never experienced much feeling in their sexual organs because their pelvic floor muscles have always been weak. Other indications of decreased sexual sensation include difficulty reaching orgasm and low or no interest in sex, although low libido is a complex issue also caused by hormonal, emotional, and other factors.

What are the risk factors for decreased sexual sensation?

The risk factors for decreased sexual sensation include all the factors that contribute to weakened pelvic floor muscles:

- Childbirth
- Chronic coughing (such as from smoking or from chronic bronchitis or asthma)
- Aging (specifically menopause)
- Obesity
- Diabetes
- Steroid use
- Smoking
- Sports injuries
- Lack of pelvic exercise (for those with naturally weak pelvic floor muscles)
- Life stress

When should I contact a doctor about decreased sexual sensation?

Sex should be a pleasurable activity. As soon as you notice any symptoms, such as lack of sensation in your sex organs or lack of interest in sex, you should consider raising the subject with your doctor, such as your obstetrician-gynecologist or urologist. Depending on your specific situation, your doctor may refer you to a physical therapist, sex therapist, or other kind of specialist. It's important for you to raise the issue with your doctor since 91 percent of health care providers do not regularly ask their patients whether they are experiencing sexual difficulty, according to the Women's Sexual Health Survey by the Women's Sexual Health Foundation.[21] You have to be proactive and ask your doctor for help when you need it.

Will my decreased sexual sensation worsen over time?

Like any muscle that is weak or has been damaged, without therapy, your pelvic floor muscles will not become stronger or heal. If you experience decreased sexual sensation, you should definitely seek therapy to address the situation. Treat your pelvic floor muscles as you would any visible muscle in your body. For instance, if you strained a muscle in your leg, you would take action to heal, rehabilitate, and strengthen the muscle. The same principle applies to the muscles in your pelvic floor, even though you can't see them.

Can decreased sexual sensation be cured?

If your decreased sexual sensation is the result of weak pelvic floor muscles, physical therapy and other exercises that strengthen these muscles will most likely help you experience a great deal more sexual sensation. Damage to these muscles can commonly be healed by conservative physical therapy. Because sexual satisfaction is a complex topic, involving not just the pelvic floor muscles but also a woman's emotional state, hormonal changes, and many other factors, there is no guarantee that healing and strengthening these muscles will automatically produce orgasmic sexual experiences. However, improving the strength and tone of these muscles will definitely help you experience more sensation during sex, usually within six to eight weeks.

How will my doctor diagnose whether I have decreased sexual sensation?

To diagnose your condition, your doctor will most likely ask you about your symptoms, including your urological and gynecological history, your sexual history and experiences, prior surgeries and medical conditions, and medications you are taking. While the questions might seem somewhat embarrassing, answer as honestly and openly as possible. Your answers will help your doctor diagnose the nature of your condition.

If you decide to seek help, ask your primary doctor to refer you to a urologist or an obstetrician-gynecologist. This specialist will likely perform a pelvic exam to determine if your decreased sensation is the result of an anatomical issue (including weakened or damaged pelvic floor muscles), a hormonal problem, or another cause.

What are my conservative treatment options for decreased sexual sensation?

There are four main conservative treatments for decreased sexual sensation that results from weakened or damaged pelvic floor muscles:

1. At-home pelvic floor retraining
2. Pelvic floor retraining guided by a specialist
3. Behavior modification and weight management
4. Medication

At-home pelvic floor retraining. Many women who experience decreased sexual sensation find the at-home retraining option attractive, since they can do these exercises in private. Chapter 7 of this book gives you a complete at-home retraining program that you can learn and do by yourself. If you choose this option, you will need to take two main steps, which we will walk you through in chapter 7:

1. Test your pelvic floor tone.
2. Tone your pelvic floor muscles.

Toning your pelvic floor muscles has many advantages:

- Studies show that postpartum women who perform pelvic floor exercises experience an improvement in sexual desire and reach more powerful orgasms with greater ease.[22]
- Nonorgasmic women with poor pelvic muscle tone who exercise these muscles experience improved sexual desire and performance, including achieving orgasm.[23]
- After age 40, women lose muscle at a rate of half a pound per year; after menopause, that rate increases to one pound per year. This loss also affects internal muscles, like pelvic floor muscles, which can lead to diminished sexual satisfaction if these muscles are weakened. Healthy pelvic floor muscles, kept in good shape with exercises, contribute to sexual pleasure and satisfaction.[24]
- Pelvic floor rehabilitation contributes to sexual satisfaction (including desire, arousal, lubrication, and orgasm) in women who experience urinary leakage during sexual activity.[25]
- Women who perform pelvic floor muscle exercises score significantly better on sexual satisfaction surveys than their counterparts who do not do exercises.[26]

Pelvic floor retraining guided by a specialist. If you know you should do pelvic floor muscle exercises, but you don't have a clear idea of how to do them, don't worry. Many women don't. One study showed that at least 50 percent of women do not properly contract their pelvic floor muscles with just written or verbal instructions.[27] Part of the problem is that you can't see these muscles. It's much easier to know if you are flexing the correct muscles when you can see them, such as when you flex the bicep muscle in your arm.

If the at-home pelvic floor retraining program leaves you confused, you may want to opt for help from a specialist, such as a physical therapist or physician. These specialists use various tools to give you positive feedback when you correctly contract your pelvic floor muscles. For instance, some will use electrical biofeedback units. Others might recommend using a pelvic floor weight, which is a plastic cone into which small weights can be placed. By inserting and holding the weight in your vagina, you strengthen your pelvic floor muscles. Still other specialists will use a manual approach, placing their fingers in or around the vaginal opening, which allows them to not only test the strength of your pelvic floor muscles, but also give you feedback when you contract the correct muscles.

Read more in chapter 8 about pelvic floor retraining guided by a specialist.

Behavior modification and weight management. In addition to strengthening your pelvic floor muscles using retraining exercises, either at home or guided by a specialist, you can address any lifestyle habits that might be putting pressure on your pelvic muscles. For instance, if you smoke and have a chronic smoker's cough, the constant strain of coughing will continue to weaken the muscles in your pelvic region. If you are carrying a few extra pounds, you might consider some weight management solutions to alleviate the pressure on your pelvic floor. Studies show that losing just a few pounds can significantly lighten the load on those muscles, as demonstrated by overweight women who have experienced reduced incontinence symptoms after weight loss.[28]

Learn more about each of these lifestyle modification techniques in chapter 8.

Medication. The primary medication prescribed to treat decreased sexual sensation is transvaginal estrogen. This medication is particularly useful for postmenopausal women, who experience decreased estrogen production, which contributes to thinning of the urethral, vaginal, and bladder lining. Estrogen has been shown to rejuvenate tissues in these areas while improving blood flow to and nerve function in the vagina. Little scientific data support the effectiveness of this therapy, but women who use transvaginal estrogen report an improvement in symptoms, including an increase in vaginal lubrication during sex.[29]

Learn more about transvaginal estrogen in chapter 8.

What are my surgical treatment options for decreased sexual sensation?

If your specialist determines that you are experiencing decreased sexual sensation as a result of a pelvic organ prolapse, which means that certain pelvic organs are bulging into other organs, then you will probably need surgery to correct the problem. Surgeries to correct pelvic organ prolapse are discussed in chapter 9.

For more information about decreased sexual sensation, see the additional resources at the end of the book.

7

At-Home Pelvic Floor Muscle Exercise Program

If you think Kegels don't work, think again. If you don't know how to do an effective pelvic floor muscle contraction (Kegel exercise), don't worry—you can learn. If you want to tone your pelvic floor muscles to improve urinary incontinence, reduce symptoms of pelvic organ prolapse, or increase sexual sensation, rest assured that you can.

Pelvic floor muscle exercise is an effective conservative therapy for all of the above conditions and is usually the first-line treatment. It definitely strengthens the pelvic floor muscles and is virtually free of side effects.[1]

Why Pelvic Floor Muscle Exercise Programs Sometimes Fail

If you have been doing exercises for your pelvic floor muscles, like Kegels, but have had unsatisfactory results, you may think that these exercises don't work. They do, but here's the catch: these exercises work only if they are done correctly and are appropriate for your current level of muscle fitness. If these exercises have not worked for you in the past, you may be encountering these common problems:

- Unable to locate the correct muscles: Studies reveal that more than 50 percent of women cannot locate and engage the correct muscles for a pelvic floor muscle contraction when given only written instructions.[2]

- Cannot do a voluntary contraction: More than 30 percent of women are unable to contract their pelvic floor muscles even after individual instruction with a therapist.[3] This may be due to lack of sensation or lack of strength in the pelvic floor muscles.
- Lack of pelvic muscle strength: Women with weakened muscles in their pelvic region tend to contract thigh, gluteal, or abdominal muscles (called overflow muscles) instead, which is ineffective for strengthening the pelvic floor muscles.[4]
- Lack of motivation: Although most women start out with high initial motivation for their pelvic exercise program, studies show that most women don't continue to follow the program after the initial treatment period (usually eight to twelve weeks). This leads to a lack of symptom improvement or the return of symptoms thought to have been cured.[5]
- Worsening symptoms: Some women do pelvic floor muscle contractions incorrectly. These women actually push down and out on their pelvic floor while doing a contraction rather than drawing the muscles inward and upward. This pushing movement is called a Valsalva maneuver, and it can worsen symptoms of urinary incontinence, pelvic organ prolapse, and decreased sexual sensation.[6]

With all these potential problems getting in the way of doing these exercises correctly, it is little wonder that controversy exists over whether Kegels and similar exercises are effective as therapy.

A Pelvic Floor Muscle Exercise Program That Works

All the problems that interfere with the effectiveness of pelvic floor muscle exercises highlight the need for a pelvic floor exercise program that:

1. Helps you locate and engage the correct muscles
2. Offers exercises appropriate to your current level of pelvic floor muscle strength

3. Motivates you to continue with exercises to resolve symptoms over the long term

With the program described in this chapter, we aim to achieve all three of these goals. Through this simple program that you do just *once per day*, you will learn step by step how to isolate and engage the correct muscles and create a customized program geared to your level of fitness.

Some exercise programs have you do up to 200 repetitions and five exercise sessions per day. For a busy woman, this kind of exercise regimen is hardly realistic. That's why we focus on helping you create a program that you do just once daily but at maximum intensity. Exercise science research shows that exercising at maximum intensity for your current level of muscle fitness, rather than doing a high number of repetitions, is needed to build muscle strength.[7]

With this kind of program, you can exercise at your convenience and make the most out of each exercise session. Our goal is for you to strengthen your pelvic floor muscles by exercising 15 minutes or less per day. We also offer many troubleshooting tips to help you get the most out of your exercise program. But before we dive into the specifics of creating a customized program for you, let's look at the scientific basis for our program.

Pelvic Floor Muscle Exercises Really Are Effective

Our exercise program is based on science, which demonstrates two facts: one, when done correctly, these exercises do strengthen the muscles of the pelvic floor;[8] and two, stronger pelvic floor muscles can relieve symptoms of urinary incontinence, pelvic organ prolapse, and decreased sexual sensation.

Stress urinary incontinence

Women with stress incontinence who follow a pelvic floor muscle exercise program have an average cure rate of 73 percent; when paired with other conservative therapies, like behavior modifications (bladder training, changes to diet, smoking cessation), the average rate of cure goes up to 97 percent.[9]

Overactive bladder and urge urinary incontinence

Women with urge incontinence or overactive bladder also show improvement after participating in a pelvic floor exercise program. For these women, the exercise program reduces the feeling of urgency as well as the number of incontinence episodes per day and voids per night.[10]

Pelvic organ prolapse

Pelvic floor muscle exercise programs are also effective for women with pelvic organ prolapse. Studies show that women with prolapse who follow this kind of exercise program have less severe symptoms, and that these exercises delay the onset of prolapse.[11] Research also shows that a pelvic exercise program increases muscle volume, shortens muscle length, and elevates the resting position of the bladder and rectum, all important benefits in a woman whose pelvic organs are no longer in the correct anatomical position.[12]

Decreased sexual sensation

In terms of sexual sensation and satisfaction, women who do pelvic floor muscle exercises score better on sexual satisfaction surveys than women who don't do pelvic floor exercises.[13] Postpartum women who use this kind of exercise program feel more sexual desire and reach orgasms more easily.[14] For women who experience urinary incontinence during intercourse, following pelvic floor exercises increases their sexual satisfaction and decreases urinary leakage.[15] Non-orgasmic women show improved sexual desire and are able to more easily achieve orgasm after doing these kinds of exercises.[16]

Clearly pelvic floor muscle exercises, when correctly done at a level appropriate to a woman's current pelvic muscle strength, can improve and sometimes cure the pelvic floor conditions we discuss in this book. In this chapter we introduce you to a program that not only will help you do correct pelvic floor muscle contractions, but will also be geared to your current level of pelvic muscle fitness. The program will become more challenging as your level of fitness increases.

The ultimate goal

The ultimate goal of this program is to help you achieve strong resting pelvic floor muscle tone. If you don't know exactly what this means, since your pelvic muscles are not visible, consider this analogy with your leg muscles. Look at your leg muscles when your legs are at rest. Are the muscles strong and toned, or do they look a bit flabby and out of shape? If your legs are a bit out of shape, you could certainly make them appear toned by flexing your leg muscles. But the goal of this program is to develop good *resting* muscle tone. If your legs look toned and fit at rest, then they have the same level of tone we aim to help you achieve with your pelvic floor muscles.

Muscles that are toned when at rest support the body. For instance, toned thigh muscles allow you to climb stairs without putting excess pressure on your knees because those muscles support your knee joints. Similarly, pelvic muscles that are toned when at rest support the bladder, uterus, and other pelvic organs, which prevents problems like urinary incontinence, pelvic organ prolapse, and decreased sexual satisfaction.

Pelvic Floor Muscle Exercise Program Requirements

To help you get the most out of the exercise program described in this chapter, we need to first review two program requirements. These requirements make sure that you are able to do a correct pelvic floor muscle contraction (or troubleshoot problems if you can't) and that the program does not interfere with any other physical conditions you may have. To maximize the benefits of this program, you must meet these requirements:

1. Be willing to touch yourself in the pelvic area. At different points in this program, we will ask you to touch your pelvic floor muscles to feel whether they are actively engaged. This touching can include placing one or two fingers in your vagina to test the strength of your pelvic contraction. Touching is also an important tool for learning to do a correct contraction, especially if you have weak pelvic floor muscles or you do not have much sensation in your pelvic region. Although this might seem embarrassing at first, remember that a pelvic floor exercise program, done correctly, can improve or even cure the conditions discussed in this book. Consider whether freedom from one or more of these conditions is worth the price of a little embarrassment.

2. Have permission from your doctor if you are currently under the care of a physician for a specific medical condition. Although these exercises are generally considered to have few to no side effects, it is always best to check with your doctor first if you have an existing medical condition. The more advanced parts of this program include movements such as marching, jogging, skipping, and lunging. If you are unsure whether you can safely perform these movements, check with your doctor before proceeding with these parts of the program.

That's it. Those are the only two requirements for the pelvic exercise program described in this book. If you are ready and willing to meet these requirements, then proceed to the next section, in which we describe how to do a correct pelvic floor muscle contraction.

How to Do a Correct Pelvic Floor Muscle Contraction

As we noted previously, many women do pelvic exercises incorrectly and end up thinking that these exercises are not an effective therapy for their urinary incontinence, pelvic organ prolapse, or decreased sexual sensation. To avoid that problem, the first step in our exercise program teaches you how to do a correct pelvic floor muscle contraction. Without the ability to locate and engage the correct muscles, you will find little benefit in the later steps of this program. A correct contraction is the foundation of an effective pelvic floor exercise program, so take as much time as you need to do the exercise below.

1. For this test, it is helpful for you to be dressed in your underwear or other thin clothing so that you can easily feel the contraction through your clothes. Wash your hands before you begin. Then, lie face up on your bed or on the floor with your legs straight and relaxed.

2. Place one hand under one buttock, slightly toward the outside edge, so that you can feel if your buttock muscle contracts. Your goal is to do a pelvic floor muscle contraction without tightening your buttock muscles.

3. Place two fingertips of your other hand between your legs in the space between your vagina and your rectum (this area is called the perineum). With the fingertips of this hand you will be able to feel your pelvic floor muscles tighten as you contract them.

4. Now contract your pelvic floor muscles, those figure 8 muscles that surround the vaginal and anal openings. If you aren't sure how to do this, imagine that you are in a crowded elevator and have gas. Contract your muscles as you would to prevent passing gas. Those are your pelvic floor muscles. Ideally, as these muscles contract, you should feel them pulling inward slightly. At the same time, be sure your buttock muscles stay relaxed. Now release the contraction.

5. Repeat this exercise, placing your hand on your abdomen. As you do the contraction, be sure that your abdominal muscles do not push outward. Release the contraction.

6. Repeat this exercise, this time placing your hand on your inner thigh. Keep the muscles of your inner thigh relaxed as you contract your pelvic floor muscles. Again, release the contraction.

If you were able to contract your pelvic floor muscles without tightening your buttocks, abdomen, or inner thighs, then you have just done a correct pelvic floor contraction. Congratulations. You are now ready to move into the testing phase of the program.

Testing Phase: Test the Strength of Your Pelvic Floor Muscles

One of the keys to success in using a pelvic floor muscle exercise program is to tailor the program to your current level of muscle fitness. A customized program empowers you to be successful and see progressive improvement without overworking your pelvic muscles or forcing you to use the incorrect muscles. This testing phase allows you to determine your current level of pelvic floor fitness in terms of the strength of your contraction, the amount of time you can hold the contraction, and the number of repetitions in a row you can perform correctly. The results will be recorded on your score card (figure 7.1) and will be the basis of your initial exercise program.

Step 1: Prepare for testing

As you perform the tests in the next steps, you'll need to record the results on the score card. Eventually, you will build a customized pelvic exercise program based on your score card. To prepare for the testing phase:

1. Make a copy of the score card and have a pen ready.
2. Be sure you have enough time and privacy so that you can feel comfortable and avoid rushing through the testing. You will need 15 to 30 minutes to complete this test.
3. Decide whether you will do the testing yourself or want your partner to perform the testing with you. Testing involves inserting a finger into your vagina and squeezing your pelvic floor muscles around the finger. If you are not comfortable using your own finger, ask your partner to help you with the assessment. Note: The same person who does the initial testing will need to do the monthly retesting as well.

Pelvic Floor Muscle Contraction (PFMC)

SCORE CARD

PFMC Test Date
_____

Section 1
POSITION →

Circle the position that allows you to perform the strongest PFMC.

Supine
(legs straight)

Side-Lying
(with bent knees)

Section 2
STRENGTH →

Did you have to use overflow muscles?

Yes   **No**

Circle the strength of your PFMC.

0   1   2   3   4

Section 3
TIME →

Note the length of time that you are able to hold a correct PFMC for one repetition.

_____ **seconds**

Section 4
REPETITIONS →

Note the number of _____-second PFMCs that you are able to perform.

_____ **repetitions**

FIGURE 7.1. Pelvic floor muscle contraction (PFMC) score card

4. Undress from the waist down.
5. Whoever will be doing the testing should wash hands thoroughly.

Step 2: Position yourself for testing

There are two positions you can use to test your muscles: supine and side-lying with bent knees.

- Supine: Lie face up on your bed or on the floor with your legs straight and relaxed (see figure 7.2).
- Side-lying with bent knees: Lie on your side on your bed or on the floor with your knees comfortably bent (see figure 7.3).

Start in the supine position for testing. If you or your partner cannot feel a noticeable contraction during testing, try the second position, side-lying with bent knees.

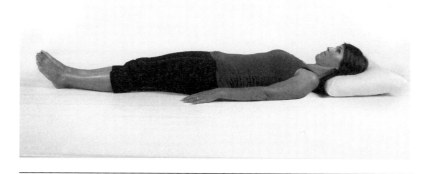

FIGURE 7.2. Supine

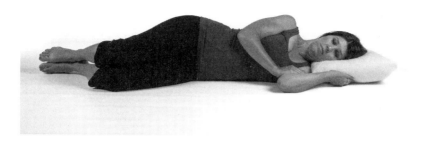

FIGURE 7.3. Side-lying with bent knees

Step 3: Test the strength of your pelvic floor muscle contraction

In this phase of testing you or your partner will gauge the strength of your contraction. You will need to record the result of this test on the score card. To perform this test:

1. Start in the supine position, lying face up on your bed or on the floor with your legs straight and relaxed, slightly spread.
2. After washing your hands, insert your index finger in your vaginal opening or have your partner insert an index finger. If inserting your finger is painful, your pelvic floor muscles may be too tight. Stop the testing phase and make an appointment with a urologist or an obstetrician-gynecologist for a thorough checkup. Proceed with this home program only if your doctor gives you permission after your exam.
3. Perform a correct pelvic floor muscle contraction according to the instructions in the above section called "How to Do a Correct Pelvic Floor Muscle Contraction." As you do the contraction, be sure that your abdominal, thigh, and buttock muscles (called overflow muscles) remain relaxed. You may need to place your hand on these muscles to ensure that you are relaxed. If

you tighten any of these muscles while doing the contraction, release the contraction and relax. Then perform the strength test again, this time keeping the overflow muscles relaxed.

If you are able to do a contraction without using your overflow muscles, circle "No" in Section 2 of your score card, in answer to the question "Did you have to use overflow muscles?" If you are unable to do a contraction without using your overflow muscles, circle "Yes" in Section 2 of your score card, then rate your contraction as 1 in the next part of this step. Do not change your rating to above 1 as you work your way through the program until you can do at least a weak contraction without using your overflow muscles. As you strengthen your pelvic muscles, you will be able to do pelvic floor muscle contractions in isolation, without the help of the overflow muscles.

4. Now rate the strength of your contraction, or have your partner rate you, according to this scale:

   0—*no* tightening felt around finger

   1—a *flicker* of a contraction felt around finger, *or* a contraction using overflow muscles

   2—a *weak* contraction felt around finger but no inward pull or upward lift* of finger

   3—a *moderate* contraction felt around finger along with a slight inward and/or upward lift of finger

   4—a *strong* contraction felt around finger with a strong inward pull and upward lift of finger

   Note: If your contraction is strong enough to have an inward pull, you or your partner will feel the finger being pulled into the vagina. Similarly, with the upward lift, the finger will be slightly lifted toward the pubic bone.

5. Record your results in Section 2 of your score card, take a breather, and move on to the next step. If you scored a 1 or higher on this test, circle the "Supine" option in Section 1 of your score card. If your score for this test was 0, read the troubleshooting advice that follows.

Troubleshooting the 0 strength contraction. If you scored a 0 on the contraction strength test, you can try to generate a stronger response by pressing the index finger slightly downward into the vaginal wall, as if stretching the vagina down toward the anal opening. This movement should increase the sensation in your vagina, and as you feel this sensation you may be able to do a stronger pelvic floor muscle contraction.

You can also change positions, from supine to side-lying with bent knees. In this position you are not fighting the force of gravity and may be more able to perform a noticeable contraction. Women with weaker muscles often find this position useful in the beginning. If this position works for you, circle the "Side-Lying" option in Section 1 of your score card.

If neither of these techniques changes your score from a 0 to at least a 1, then we recommend that you consult a doctor specializing in urology or obstetrics/gynecology before proceeding with this program.

Step 4: Test how long you can hold a pelvic floor muscle contraction

Remain in the same position for this next test. If you changed from supine to side-lying with bent knees during the previous test, remain in that position. For this test, follow the same instructions as for testing the strength of your contraction but instead of noting the strength of your contraction, determine the amount of time you can hold a correct contraction (up to 10 seconds).

Be sure that your overflow muscles (abdominal, thigh, and buttock muscles) remain relaxed throughout the entire contraction. If you feel any of these muscles tighten during your contraction, stop counting seconds. The tightening of overflow muscles tells you that your pelvic floor muscles are beginning to tire and that you are no longer doing a correct contraction.

If you are unable to hold a contraction without using your overflow muscles, don't worry. Simply put "2 seconds" in Section 3 of your score card. This means you will start out with 2-second contractions when you begin your exercise program. If you were able to hold a contraction without using your overflow muscles, record that time in Section 3 of your score card. Then write the number of seconds in the first blank in Section 4 of your score card. Rest for a short time before moving on to the next step.

Step 5: Test how many pelvic floor muscle contraction repetitions you can perform

This final step helps you determine the number of times you can perform a correct contraction.

1. Note the time you recorded in Section 3 of your score card. This was the longest you could hold a correct contraction.
2. Now do the maximum number of correct contractions you can up to 10 repetitions. Hold each contraction as long as you did in the previous step, and rest for 10 seconds between contractions. For instance, if the longest you could hold a contraction in the previous step was 5 seconds, in this step you will perform as many 5-second contractions you can (up to 10 times), with a 10-second rest period between each contraction.

   Be sure to stop counting repetitions as soon as you feel your overflow muscles start to tighten or when you can no longer hold your contraction for the required length of time. If you cannot do a pelvic floor muscle contraction without using your overflow muscles, then do the maximum number of 2-second contractions you can, with 10-second rest periods, while using your overflow muscles.

Record the number of repetitions in Section 4 of your score card and rest.

Congratulations. You have completed the testing phase of the program. You can now move forward to designing the first phase of your own customized pelvic floor muscle exercise program.

The Five F's of a Fit Pelvic Floor

The exercise program in this chapter has five parts, arranged in order of progressive difficulty. This stepwise progression allows you to focus first on strengthening your pelvic muscle exercises in isolation, and then to incorporate pelvic floor muscle contractions into your daily life. Each part begins with the letter F. The five F's are listed below and described beginning on page 107.

F#1. Focused and fast: Shows you how to strengthen your pelvic floor muscles in isolation. Teaches you how to do short quick contractions in addition to the longer holds.

F#2. Functional: Teaches you how to pre-contract your pelvic floor muscles before stressful activities like coughing. This part also incorporates pelvic floor muscle contractions in daily activities, such as changing positions, walking, stepping up, and squatting.

F#3. Freedom: Integrates contractions with more vigorous activities, including marching, skipping, jumping, and jogging.

F#4. Fun: Brings contractions into the bedroom for more satisfying sexual experiences.

F#5. Future: Helps you create a maintenance program to keep your pelvic floor muscles fit if you decide to return to a high-impact sport.

During the entire program you will be recording your efforts, progress, and the status of your symptoms in a journal. A sample journal is shown in figure 7.4 (figure 7.5 is a blank page for you to use).

Frequently Asked Questions about the Five F's Program

Before starting the Five F's program, please read the responses to frequently asked questions that follow. This information may answer questions you have as you proceed through the program and can help you get the most out of each part of the program.

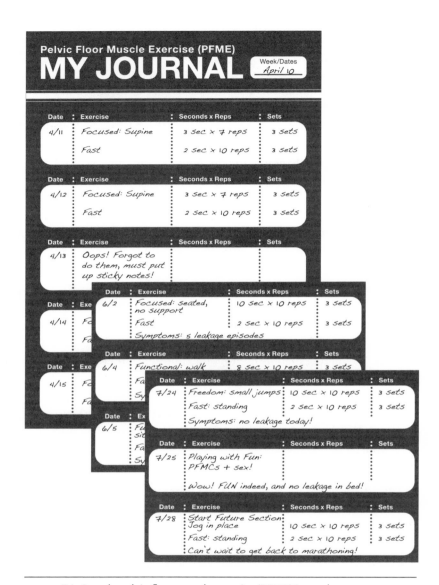

FIGURE 7.4. Sample pelvic floor muscle exercise (PFME) journal

How much time should I spend in each part of the program?

There is no way to easily answer this question for every woman who participates in this program, since the length of time spent on each part depends on each person's current level of muscle fitness. But most women will spend between three and five weeks on each part. Don't worry if you spend more or less time. Just proceed at your own pace. As long as you can complete the exercises in each part correctly, go ahead and proceed to the next part.

When can I expect to see results from this program?

Depending on your level of pelvic floor fitness, you might see results, such as symptom improvement or an increase in pelvic floor muscle strength, within just a few weeks. According to research in the exercise science field, women doing a program like ours usually gain maximum strength after about five months.[17] But you might not be seeking the maximum strength necessary to run a marathon or kickbox without leaking urine.

If you just want to be able to run errands or pick up your baby without urinary incontinence, you probably won't need five months to achieve your results. The length of time needed to achieve results depends mostly on your ultimate goals and your ability to stick with the program.

How can I help myself remember to do the program every day?

This is an important question because one of the main reasons women don't get the results they hope for is that they don't consistently follow the exercise program. Fortunately, there are multiple tricks for remembering to do your exercises daily:

- Do your exercises at the same time each day, such as first thing in the morning or right before you go to bed.

- Get an exercise buddy and motivate each other. You and your buddy can call each other at an agreed-on time to remind each other. Knowing that another person knows you have committed to a daily program is an excellent motivator.
- Set an alarm on your smart phone, computer, or kitchen timer to remind you to exercise.
- Put up sticky notes all through the house and in your car as reminders.
- Get a group of women together to exercise. Studies show that exercise groups can be effective.[18] You may not meet every day, but being part of a group can motivate you to do your exercises on the days you don't meet.

What if I miss a day or two of the exercise program? Should I double up?

If you miss a day, or even a few days, of your exercise program you don't need to double up your repetitions. Instead, focus on the reasons you skipped days in your program. Then try to address those problems, either with better reminders or better scheduling. Don't worry. Your muscles won't lose condition during that time. Studies from exercise science suggest that exercising one to two times weekly at high intensity is enough to maintain muscle strength.[19] When you miss days your muscles will maintain condition, although you will not be increasing muscle strength. Just don't miss more than a day or two, since the same studies show that stopping the exercises for even a week can lead to a 5 to 10 percent reduction in muscle strength.[20]

How often should I repeat the testing phase to check my progress?

In the program, you will be asked to retest your muscle strength at the end of each of the five parts. If you find yourself spending more than a month in a particular part, however, retest yourself once a month. For consistency, remember to have the same person who tested you initially (you or your partner) retest you each time.

Why does the program suggest I fill out a daily journal?

A daily journal is important because it tracks your efforts and your progress in a visible way. With any exercise program, it is common to make progress but not notice it. This is even more likely with a pelvic floor exercise program, since your pelvic floor muscles are not visible, so you won't be able to see increases in muscle volume and tone. By keeping a daily journal, you get the positive feedback of seeing a long list of your efforts, all the repetitions you have done to date. You also notice daily differences in symptoms, such as a slight decrease in urinary incontinence episodes over the span of a week. While the decrease in symptoms may be slight, it is nevertheless forward progress. Any forward progress motivates you to keep going with the exercise program. So jot down as much detail as you can to make your daily journal an asset in your program.

F#1. Focused and Fast Pelvic Floor Muscle Contractions

The information in this part will help you create a customized program in which you begin by toning your pelvic floor muscles in isolation. The goal of practicing pelvic floor muscle contractions in isolation is to give you plenty of practice engaging the correct pelvic muscles, until a correct contraction becomes almost automatic. In this part, you will also learn how to do fast contractions. After you create your customized baseline program (Step 1), perform this program daily, proceeding to the next steps as directed, until you are able to complete Step 5.

Step 1: Create your baseline program

Referring to your score card from the testing phase, create your baseline exercise program by using the following data from your test: position, seconds you held a contraction, and number of repetitions you performed correctly. Using that information, create your program using this formula:

Once a day, do your pelvic floor muscle contractions as follows:

- Strongest position: Do the contractions in either supine or side-lying with bent knees (whichever you circled on your score card).
- Time: Hold each contraction for the maximum length of time you held it during the test.
- Repetitions: Do the maximum number of repetitions you could correctly do during the test, with a 10-second rest between each repetition.
- Rest for one minute, and then do two more sets with a one-minute rest in between.

For example, suppose this is the information you gathered during the testing phase:

- Position: You were not able to feel a contraction in the supine position, but you could feel a flicker in the side-lying with bent knees position.
- Time: The longest you could hold a correct contraction was three seconds.
- Repetitions: The most correct contractions you could perform in a row was seven.

You would use this information to create the following customized program to be done once daily:

Three sets of the following with a one-minute rest between sets:

- Perform contractions in the side-lying with bent knees position.
- Hold each contraction for 3 seconds, with a 10-second rest in between.
- Do seven repetitions per set.

Once you have practiced this baseline program for a day or two, proceed to Step 2, where you will add fast pelvic floor muscle contractions to your daily program.

Pelvic Floor Muscle Exercise (PFME)
MY JOURNAL

Week/Dates
_____

Date	Exercise	Seconds x Reps	Sets

Date	Exercise	Seconds x Reps	Sets

Date	Exercise	Seconds x Reps	Sets

Date	Exercise	Seconds x Reps	Sets

Date	Exercise	Seconds x Reps	Sets

FIGURE 7.5. Blank journal page

Tip: Use copies of the blank journal page provided in figure 7.5 to start keeping a log of your daily program efforts. Simply fill in the date, exercise details, number of sets and repetitions you performed, and the amount of time you held each contraction. As you progress through the program, also jot down any changes or improvements in your symptoms or general health. Keep your journal pages where you can easily see them because they can remind you to do your program daily.

Step 2: Add fast pelvic floor muscle contractions

The contractions you have been performing so far, with relatively long hold times for each contraction, will strengthen the "slow twitch" muscle fibers, also called "marathoner" fibers. These fibers hold your pelvic organs in place and support them throughout the day.

Your pelvic floor muscles also have "fast twitch" muscle fibers (or "sprinter" muscle fibers), which are the ones that react quickly to tighten the muscles around the urethra and support your pelvic organs when you sneeze, lift, or do any activity that suddenly increases your intra-abdominal pressure. To truly strengthen your pelvic floor muscles, you need to exercise both the slow twitch and the fast twitch muscle fibers.

To exercise the fast twitch muscle fibers, you need to add fast contractions to your daily program. To do fast contractions, simply perform three sets of the following with a one-minute rest between sets:

- Get into the same position you have been in to perform the longer duration contractions.
- Hold each contraction for two seconds, with a two-second rest in between. The resting phase is very important.
- Do 10 repetitions per set.

Add these fast contractions to your daily baseline program within a day or two of starting Step 1. Record the fast pelvic floor muscle contractions in your daily journal.

Step 3: Maximize your time and repetitions

Once you feel comfortable performing your baseline program, work on improving your contractions from Step 1. Focus on increasing the amount of time you hold each contraction and the number of repetitions you perform in each set.

At this stage your goal is to be able to hold each pelvic floor muscle contraction for 10 seconds, perform 10 repetitions per set, and complete three sets.

Remember to keep your contractions correct. If you increase your hold time or repetitions but find that your overflow muscles are taking over, decrease the hold time or repetitions until you can once again do correct contractions. Experiment with hold times and repetitions as your pelvic floor muscles become stronger, balancing correct contractions with ever increasing hold times and repetitions.

Continue doing your fast contractions throughout the rest of the program.

Step 4: Perform the tampon tug

When you are able to achieve the goal stated in Step 3, the next step is to perform the tampon tug. The tampon tug measures whether your contractions are strong enough to hold a tampon in place as you try to gently pull it out. To perform the tampon tug, wash your hands thoroughly, undress from the waist down, and have a tampon in its applicator, soaked with warm water, ready.

1. Position yourself just as you do for your baseline program (either supine or side-lying with knees bent).
2. Insert the tampon in your vaginal opening, remove the applicator, and hold the string.
3. Perform a pelvic floor muscle contraction while you gently tug on the tampon string (be careful not to tighten your abdominal, thigh, or buttock muscles).

If you are able to hold the tampon in place with your contraction, congratulations. Your pelvic muscles have definitely grown strong enough for you to move on to the next and final step in F#1.

Step 5: Progress through the positions

Now that you can correctly perform three sets of 10-second contractions, with 10 repetitions per set, as well as do the tampon tug, the final step in this part is to do your baseline program in progressively more difficult positions. The positions, in order of difficulty, are:

- Side-lying with knees bent
- Supine
- Seated reclining with back support, legs straight (as on a bed leaning on pillows; see figure 7.6)
- Seated upright without back support (as on the edge of a toilet seat; see figure 7.7)

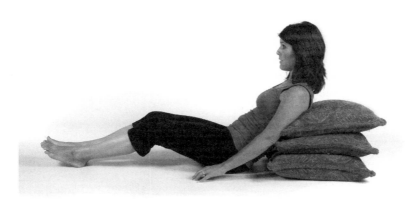

FIGURE 7.6. Seated reclining with back support

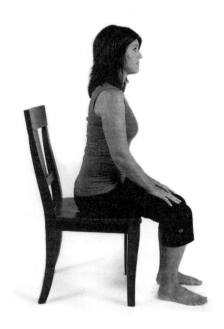

FIGURE 7.7. Seated upright without back support

To progress through the positions, find the position you currently use for your baseline program and move to the next position in the list. If you currently use the supine position, for example, move to the seated reclining position. If you started in the side-lying with knees bent position, move to the supine position. (Note that if you started in supine, you do not need to do side-lying with knees bent.)

Work through your baseline program in this new position until you can perform three sets of 10-second contractions, with 10 repetitions per set, as well as do the tampon tug. Move through all the positions until you can successfully perform the maximum sets, hold times, and repetitions, as well as the tampon tug. Continue doing your fast contractions as you progress through the positions, and remember to continue recording your results in your daily journal.

Once you have progressed through all the positions, you can move on to the next part, F#2, in which you will incorporate pelvic floor muscle contractions into regular daily movements.

F#2. Functional Pelvic Floor Muscle Contractions

This functional part of the program is where you really begin to reap the benefits of your exercise. In this part, you learn to integrate contractions into daily life, which will both prevent symptoms and start building your body's automatic pelvic floor muscle contraction. In other words, by learning to do contractions with normal daily occurrences, like coughing, walking, or stepping up, you will eventually teach your body to automatically do these contractions whenever your intra-abdominal pressure increases. Automatic contractions will then prevent or lessen symptoms like urinary incontinence.

Women whose pelvic floor muscles are not weakened naturally have this automatic muscle contraction response; women with weak pelvic floor muscles must relearn this natural and unconscious contraction.[21] To help you relearn the automatic muscle contraction response, we first teach you to do a conscious pelvic floor muscle contraction before an activity for which you need extra pelvic floor support, such as coughing or clearing your throat. This conscious contraction is called a "pre-contraction." Once you have mastered the pre-contraction, you then learn to do correct contractions during simple activities such as standing, walking, and lifting.

As in part F#1, continue performing the fast contractions throughout this part, but in the standing position. While standing, perform three sets of the following with a one-minute rest between sets:

- Hold each contraction for two seconds with a two-second rest in between.
- Do 10 repetitions per set.

Step 1: Learn the pre-contraction

When you perform a pre-contraction, you do the pelvic floor muscle contraction as you learned in part F#1 and add a transverse abdominal contraction for additional support. The transverse abdominus muscle, like a corset, wraps around your lower abdomen just above your pelvis. This muscle provides core stability and support. You will need the additional support of the abdominal contraction as you start doing contractions with movement. To do a pre-contraction:

1. Stand with your feet shoulder-width apart. Be sure that you are standing fully upright, with your ears, shoulders, hips, knees, and ankles in alignment (see figure 7.8).
2. Perform a contraction as you did in F#1.
3. Hold the contraction as you perform a transverse abdominal contraction as follows:
   - Exhale as you pull your belly button inward toward your spine.
   - Maintain the correct postural position, standing fully upright and in alignment, neither flattening nor overarching your spine.
   - Be sure to keep your thigh and buttock muscles relaxed.
4. Hold both the pelvic floor muscle contraction and the abdominal contraction as you clear your throat.
5. Release both contractions and relax.

Step 2: Use the pre-contraction

Now that you know how to perform a pre-contraction, practice doing it, first with throat clearing and then with coughing. Once you can easily do 5 to 10 repetitions with throat clearing, and 5 repetitions with coughing, you can move on to Step 3. If you need several days to feel comfortable with the pre-contraction, continue doing your daily program from F#1 at the same time.

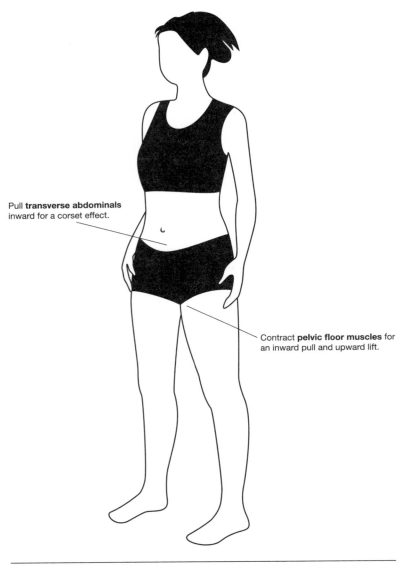

Pull **transverse abdominals** inward for a corset effect.

Contract **pelvic floor muscles** for an inward pull and upward lift.

FIGURE 7.8. Correct postural alignment for a pelvic floor muscle contraction

Step 3: Combine pelvic floor muscle contractions with movement

Now you are ready to combine the pelvic floor muscle contraction and the abdominal contraction with movement. The movements in this step are listed in order of difficulty. Use one movement per day for your pelvic floor muscle exercises, according to the instructions, until you locate the most difficult one that you can perform correctly. Then use this movement as your daily exercise program until you can progress to the next movement. Keep moving through the list until you can perform the most difficult exercise while doing correct contractions.

Hold both the pelvic contraction and the transverse abdominal contraction (we'll refer to them together as the dual contractions) while you do one of the following movements:

- Walk: Walk for 10 seconds holding the dual contractions. Release the contractions and stand and rest for 10 seconds. Repeat 9 more times for a total of 10 repetitions in a set. Perform three sets in total, with a one-minute rest between sets.
- Sit, stand, sit: Move from sitting to standing and back to sitting for 10 seconds while holding the dual contractions. Release the contractions and rest for 10 seconds. Repeat 9 more times for a total of 10 repetitions per set. Perform three sets total, with a one-minute rest between sets (see figure 7.9).
- Step up, step down: Holding the dual contractions, step up at least three inches (onto a bench or step) with one foot, and then step down. Repeat this movement for 10 seconds. Release the contractions and rest for 10 seconds. Repeat 9 more times for a total of 10 repetitions per set, alternating between your left and right feet to step up. Perform three sets total, with a one-minute rest between sets (see figure 7.10).
- Squat: Stand with your legs slightly more than shoulder-width apart. Hold the dual contractions and squat down as far as your joints can comfortably tolerate, then rise to standing.

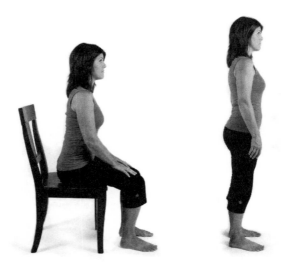

FIGURE 7.9. Sit to stand

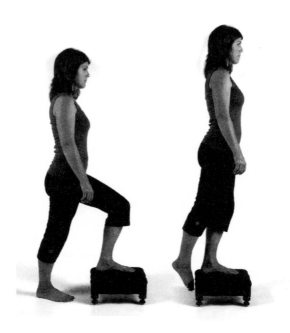

FIGURE 7.10. Step up, step down

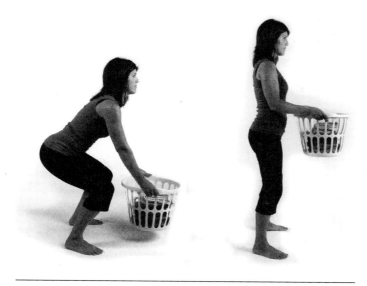

FIGURE 7.11. Lift

Repeat this movement for 10 seconds. Release the contractions and rest for 10 seconds. Repeat 9 more times for a total of 10 repetitions per set. Perform three sets total, with a one-minute rest between sets.

- Lift: Holding the dual contractions, squat down and pick up a light object, like a book, and then stand back up. Squat down and put the item back down on the floor. Repeat this movement for 10 seconds. Release the contractions and rest for 10 seconds. Repeat 9 more times for a total of 10 repetitions per set. Perform three sets total, with a one-minute rest between sets (see figure 7.11).

Remember to keep track of your progress and results in your journal pages. Stay with this part until you can do the most difficult movement while correctly holding the dual contractions and can do the fast contractions in the standing position. At this point you might also contemplate enrolling in a Pilates or yoga class to continue to build your core strength, which will only enhance the effect of your pelvic floor muscle contractions.

If you are satisfied at this point with your progress, you can skip to F#5, which helps you create a maintenance program. By doing a maintenance program, you keep your pelvic muscles toned and strong as well as keeping any symptoms under control. If you are an athlete or want to return to a more active lifestyle, which might include activities like aerobics or running, proceed to the next part.

F#3. Freedom Pelvic Floor Muscle Contractions

In F#3, you move beyond simply integrating pelvic contractions into basic movements. As the name of this part implies, the goal of these exercises is to free you to really move, with marching, skipping, lunging, and more.

These exercises are arranged from least to most difficult. Use one movement per day for your pelvic exercises according to the instructions until you locate the most difficult one that you can perform correctly. Then use this movement as your daily exercise program until you can progress to the next exercise. Keep moving through the list until you can perform the most difficult exercise while doing correct contractions. Depending on your level of fitness and your athletic goals, in this part of the program, you can do *up* to three sets per exercise session.

Hold both the pelvic contraction and the transverse abdominal contraction (the dual contractions) while you do one of the following movements:

- March in place: March in place for 10 seconds holding the dual contractions. Release the contractions and rest in place for 10 seconds. Repeat 9 more times for a total of 10 repetitions in a set. Perform up to three sets total with a one-minute rest between sets.
- Skip: Skip for 10 seconds holding the dual contractions. Release the contractions and rest in place for 10 seconds. Repeat

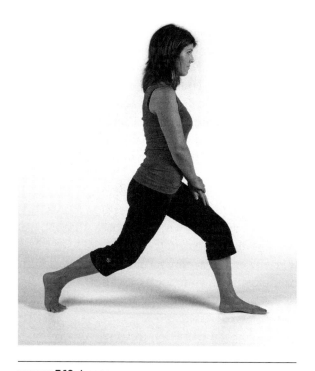

FIGURE 7.12. Lunge

9 more times for a total of 10 repetitions in a set. Perform up to three sets total with a one-minute rest between sets.

- Lunge: Holding the dual contractions, stand with your feet shoulder-width apart, and then take a large step forward with your right leg. Hold onto a chair for support if necessary and bend both knees as far as you comfortably can. Then straighten both legs. Continue to bend and straighten your legs for 10 seconds. Rest in place for 10 seconds. Repeat 9 more times for a total of 10 repetitions in a set. Perform up to three sets total with a one-minute rest between sets. Alternate the forward leg with each set to ensure you work both sides of your body equally (see figure 7.12).

- Small jumps: Perform small jumps in place for 10 seconds, using both legs to push off the ground and land, while holding the dual contractions. Rest in place for 10 seconds. Repeat 9 more times for a total of 10 repetitions in a set. Perform up to three sets total with a one-minute rest between sets.
- Jog in place: Hold the dual contractions while jogging in place for 10 seconds. Rest in place for 10 seconds. Repeat 9 more times for a total of 10 repetitions in a set. Perform up to three sets total with a one-minute rest between sets.

Remember to keep track of your progress and activities in your daily journal. Be sure to celebrate your achievements. If you are not sure whether you are improving, flip back through your journal pages and read your previous notes. You should see some real progress. In addition, keep up with your fast contractions in the standing position. Keep practicing your contractions in combination with the exercises in this part, as well as your fast contractions, until you can do the most difficult exercises.

At this point, you can transition to a maintenance program three times a week. For your program, choose one exercise from this part each time you exercise. To keep the exercises interesting, you might want to choose a different exercise each session. Also keep doing the fast contractions in the standing position as part of your maintenance. Read more about setting up a maintenance program in part F#5.

Then, if you are ready for a little fun in the bedroom, proceed to the next part, F#4. The exercises in F#4 are supplemental to your maintenance program.

F#4. Fun Pelvic Floor Muscle Contractions (in the Bedroom)

You have been putting a lot of effort into your pelvic floor muscle contractions, and now it's time to have fun with them—in the bedroom. In chapter 6, we described how toned and fit pelvic floor muscles can improve sexual satisfaction. Not only do strong pelvic floor muscles have increased blood flow to engorge the clitoris, but they also have more nerve endings than weak pelvic floor muscles.[22] Also, the pelvic floor muscles surround the internal parts of the clitoris—the parts you can't see—and contracting these muscles increases the blood flow and sensation of the clitoris.[23] Given that the clitoris has between six thousand and eight thousand sensory nerve endings, you can see how flexing your pelvic floor muscles to stimulate your clitoris can lead to having more fun in the bedroom.[24]

Doing pelvic floor muscle contractions in the bedroom

You can do pelvic contractions in many ways during intimate moments with your partner. Consider these five ideas for playing with your contractions.

1. Foreplay: This phase of lovemaking is a perfect time to start doing contractions. Exercising your pelvic floor muscles during foreplay will increase blood flow to your genitals and promote lubrication, which heightens arousal.[25] Experiment with quick contractions or longer holding contractions to see which arouses you the most.
2. Penetration: Perform and hold a contraction during penetration by your partner, and then relax each time he withdraws. This will increase sensation for both of you.
3. Withdrawal: Similarly, you can perform and hold a contraction each time your partner withdraws, and relax the contraction during penetration. This contraction will feel similar to the tampon tug, since you are doing a contraction against resistance, but obviously this is much more fun.
4. Quick flicks: After penetration, both you and your partner remain still while you do a series of fast contractions, also known as "quick flicks." These quick flicks can increase sexual sensation for both of you.
5. Gradual contraction: Similar to the quick flicks, both you and your partner remain still after penetration. Then you perform

a long, slow, and gradual contraction. Some men report that this gradual pelvic floor muscle contraction feels like a pelvic "ripple" and is very arousing.

Of course, these five ways of using contractions during sex are only guidelines and suggestions. Now that you have quite a bit of experience with using your pelvic floor muscles, you can explore multiple different ways to use contractions to enhance your sexual activities. Don't forget that an orgasm is a series of pelvic floor muscle contractions, so it gives you both pleasure and strength training for your pelvic muscles. Good sex truly is good for you.

F#5. Future Pelvic Floor Muscle Contractions

Most women wonder if they will have to do pelvic floor exercises for the rest of their lives. Yes, but not in the same way as you have been doing them so far. Specifically, once you have strengthened your pelvic floor muscles to your satisfaction, you will need to continue with a maintenance program for the rest of your life, but not with the same frequency. Your maintenance program will be a scaled-down version of the program you have done to this point. You should start your maintenance program once you have achieved a satisfactory improvement in symptoms, or once you are ready to return to regular sports activities.

The entire program you have been doing is based on exercise science research on regular skeletal muscles. We use principles from exercise science because pelvic floor muscles are regular skeletal muscles, just like your biceps or quadriceps, and therefore develop in the same way.[26] Exercise science research tells us that much less effort is needed to maintain muscle strength than to build it. According to studies, muscle strength maintenance requires the same intensity of exercise, but less frequently (about two times per week). In our clinical experience, doing pelvic floor muscles exercises *three* times per week is more effective and easier to remember, and that is what we recommend.

To create your own maintenance program, choose any exercise

movement you have successfully completed from F#2 or F#3. If you did not do any exercises from F#3 (the freedom part of the program), then you should choose exercises from F#2 (the functional part of the program).

Perform three sets of 10 repetitions each, with 10-second holds per repetition. Include 10 seconds of rest between repetitions and a minute of rest between sets. Also continue with the fast contractions in the standing position. Feel free to choose different movements on different days to keep your exercise program interesting. For instance, you might choose marching in place plus fast contractions on Monday, squatting plus fast contractions on Wednesday, and small jumps plus fast contractions on Friday.

Every day, continue to use pre-contractions before you sneeze, cough, or otherwise increase pressure on your bladder and pelvic floor. Research confirms that the more you practice this pre-contraction with the correct timing, the more likely your body will perform this movement as an automatic reaction.[27]

Most of all, enjoy the rewards of all your hard work in strengthening your pelvic floor muscles. Have fun in the bedroom and enjoy your newfound freedom to move, exercise, and live without worrying about pelvic floor weakness.

8

Additional Conservative Treatments

More is better when it comes to treating pelvic floor issues with conservative therapies. In chapter 7 we gave you detailed step-by-step instructions on how to strengthen and tone your pelvic floor muscles with various Kegel-type exercises. Done properly and consistently, these exercises can provide immediate relief for symptoms of urinary incontinence, decreased sexual sensation, and even pelvic organ prolapse.

Sometimes, though, pelvic floor exercises don't provide complete relief from symptoms. In these situations, the "more is better" approach really works well. Many women find that pairing pelvic floor exercises with other conservative treatments can provide greater improvement in symptoms.

For instance, women with mixed urinary incontinence often find that their symptoms improve when they combine pelvic floor muscle exercises with certain kinds of medication, which we review in this chapter. Other forms of conservative therapy that work well for mixed incontinence symptoms include diet modification and weight loss. For example, even making a minor lifestyle change such as avoiding caffeinated drinks like coffee and soda can make a big difference in urine leakage symptoms.

What's so great about conservative therapies for pelvic floor issues is that they are not complicated and are usually fairly simple to integrate into your existing lifestyle. The key to maximizing their effectiveness is perseverance. What works for one woman's pelvic floor issues may not work for another's. If you find that combining one or more conservative therapies does not create the desired improvement in your symptoms, try a different combination. For instance, if you try pairing pelvic floor muscle exercises with certain medications but are still not getting relief from your symptoms, consider combining pelvic exercises with diet modification and other lifestyle changes. These lifestyle changes may include quitting smoking, bladder retraining, and resolving issues like constipation.

With conservative treatments for pelvic floor health issues, there is no "right" answer. Instead, success with these treatments is a matter of being willing to explore different options until you find the right solution for your situation, whether you are dealing with urine leakage, decreased sexual sensation, or a combination of symptoms.

We urge you to be as persistent as you need to be, both with yourself and with your health care providers, in finding the right treatments for your symptoms. Remember, the statistics are in your favor: the Agency for Healthcare Research and Quality reports that for 8 out of 10 women with urinary incontinence, symptoms can be improved, especially when women seek help.[1] So be active, be aggressive, and be your own best health care advocate. Don't give up until you get the results you want, whether that means staying dry or being able to return to an active and healthy lifestyle.

Eight conservative treatments (seven of which are described in this chapter) are most effective for the different types of pelvic floor health issues, including urinary incontinence, pelvic organ prolapse, and decreased sexual sensation. One of the most important therapies, of course, is at-home pelvic floor retraining, as described in chapter 7. The beauty of learning how to do pelvic floor exercises is that you become an empowered advocate for your own pelvic health. Plus, you can do these exercises almost anywhere, and when they are done faithfully, they can help maintain the strength and health of your pelvic floor muscles for years to come.

For even more effective results in controlling pelvic floor issues, you might consider other conservative therapies in addition to at-home pelvic floor retraining. In this chapter, we describe each therapy, which conditions it helps, and who offers the kind of therapy, such as your doctor, a therapist, or a nurse practitioner. The therapies are listed in order, from most to least commonly prescribed.

- Pelvic floor retraining guided by a specialist
- Medication
- Behavior and diet modifications plus weight management
- Acupuncture
- Percutaneous tibial nerve stimulation
- Vaginal pessaries
- Urethral dilation

Pelvic Floor Retraining Guided by a Specialist (plus Biofeedback)

Which conditions does this therapy help?

Pelvic floor retraining, guided by a specialist, can be helpful for symptoms of stress urinary incontinence, urge urinary incontinence, mixed urinary incontinence, pelvic organ prolapse, decreased sexual sensation, and pelvic floor weakness.

Who offers this kind of therapy?

A wide variety of specialists offer pelvic floor retraining, including urologists, urogynecologists, nurses and nurse practitioners, and physical therapists. You may need to get a referral from your primary doctor to visit one of these specialists.

What is pelvic floor retraining guided by a specialist?

Pelvic floor retraining consists of several techniques designed to help you become more aware of and strengthen the muscles in your pelvic floor. Symptoms like urinary leakage, pelvic organ prolapse, and decreased sexual sensation often improve as your pelvic floor muscles grow stronger. Stronger pelvic muscles help support the bladder and urethra, which can help prevent urine leakage. Toned pelvic muscles also help hold all your pelvic organs in place, so they don't "bulge," which is what happens with pelvic organ prolapse.

The best known of these pelvic floor retraining exercises is the Kegel. We describe many variations of this exercise in the previous chapter on at-home pelvic floor retraining. Kegels strengthen your urinary sphincter and pelvic floor muscles. The benefit of Kegels is that you can do these exercises almost anywhere—while you're driving, watching television, or sitting at your desk at work.

Your specialist will do an intravaginal exam to determine the tone, strength, and endurance of your pelvic floor muscles. He or she also considers your posture, assesses your core muscle strength, and weighs the impact of daily activities on your condition. Once all these factors have been assessed, the specialist will then teach you how to locate and engage the correct pelvic floor muscles in isolation and during daily activities. This is important if you are among the 50 percent of women who cannot easily identify and contract their pelvic floor muscles by following only written instructions.[2]

Your therapist may also use biofeedback in your pelvic floor retraining program, which can give you feedback that is either visual or auditory. Most often, this involves placing an electrode on the relevant muscles. The electrodes are linked to a video screen or audio feed, which offers visual or auditory feedback when you are tightening certain muscles. This feedback helps you learn to feel the sensation of tightening these muscles. A similar approach is mild electrical stimulation—electrodes placed in the vagina or rectum for short periods stimulate the pelvic muscles to tone and strengthen them.

Another option your therapist may introduce is the vaginal weight. A vaginal weight is a plastic cone into which small weights can be placed. You insert the weight into your vagina, just as you would a tampon, and then tighten your pelvic floor muscles around the weight to hold it inside. The weights inside the cone are gradually increased as your pelvic muscles grow stronger and can hold heavier weights.

How effective is pelvic floor retraining?

Studies show that pelvic floor retraining can be an effective therapy for symptoms of pelvic floor weakness, including urinary incontinence, pelvic organ prolapse, and loss of sexual sensation. As with all types of therapy and exercise programs, success often depends on your willingness to learn to do the exercises correctly and your consistency in following the program. According to the Mayo Clinic, you should expect to see results in eight to twelve weeks, and some women experience dramatic results sooner.[3] You should expect to incorporate these exercises into your regular health regimen to keep your pelvic floor muscles strong throughout your life.

Studies show that women with stress incontinence strongly benefit from doing Kegels. A review of recent studies on the effects of Kegel exercises shows that women who did the exercises were anywhere from 2.5 to 17 times more likely to be cured of symptoms.[4] In another study, 70 percent of women with urinary incontinence who used vaginal weights saw improvement in their symptoms after four to six weeks of using them.

Medication

Which conditions does this therapy help?

Medication can alleviate symptoms of all three types of urinary incontinence (stress, urge, and mixed). Estrogen has also proven useful for some women dealing with decreased sexual sensation. This is important considering the scope of this problem. According to a 2005 study published in the *American Journal of Obstetrics and Gynecology*, sexual dysfunction affects 48 percent of women.[5]

Who offers this kind of therapy?

Your doctor or specialist will need to prescribe the medications used to treat urinary incontinence.

What kinds of medications are prescribed?

Depending on your diagnosis, your doctor or specialist may prescribe one or more medications. Here we list the most commonly prescribed drugs by their generic names for each condition. As noted in chapter 2, the medications we list for stress incontinence are not currently approved by the FDA to treat pure stress incontinence, although studies indicate that they do improve or even cure stress urinary incontinence symptoms.[6]

Drugs commonly prescribed for stress urinary incontinence

- ANTIMUSCARINIC MEDICATION. These medications are FDA approved for urge and mixed incontinence, but they commonly improve symptoms of stress incontinence as well. The drugs work by blocking the contractile receptors in the bladder and can also increase bladder capacity. Studies show that this kind of medication has a small but noticeable effect on symptoms.[7] Before prescribing these medications, your doctor will want to determine that you can empty your bladder completely. All antimuscarinics can prevent you from emptying your bladder if your bladder doesn't normally empty completely. Your bladder can be tested by ultrasound or catheterization.

  Examples of antimuscarinic drugs include darifenacin, fesoterodine, oxybutynin, solifenacin, trospium chloride, and tolterodine. Most of these medications are available in an extended-release form, and oxybutynin is also available as a skin patch and a gel.

  Side effects: The most common side effect of this class of medications is dry mouth, which you can alleviate by sucking on sugar-free candy or chewing gum to produce more saliva. You can also take small sips of water, rinse your mouth with water, or try an "artificial saliva" spray available over the counter. Do not drink excessive amounts of fluid to counteract the dryness. Some women also experience irritation with the oxybutynin skin patch or gel, which can be alleviated by changing the location of the patch or where the gel is applied.

- TRICYCLIC MEDICATION. This is an older class of drugs that is inexpensive and often prescribed for depression. In very small doses, tricyclic medication causes the bladder muscle to relax, while also causing the smooth muscles at the neck of the bladder to contract.[8] Examples of medications in this class are amitriptyline and imipramine. They must be used with caution in the very elderly.

  Side effects: The most common side effect of these medications is drowsiness, so they are often taken at night, which can also help with nighttime urinary incontinence. Amitriptyline can also cause dry mouth. See the side effects listed for antimuscarinic medications for ways to alleviate dry mouth.

- ESTROGEN. This drug works primarily by thickening the lining of the urethra. This thickening may help support the bladder and decrease symptoms of stress incontinence, especially if the hormone is used long term. Estrogen has been shown to increase blood flow, improve nerve function, and rejuvenate tissues in the urethra and vagina.

  This form of medication is prescribed primarily for postmenopausal women, since the decrease in the body's natural production of estrogen contributes to thinning of the urethral, vaginal, and bladder lining. Estrogen has also been shown to prevent urinary tract infections in postmenopausal women.[9] Although little scientific evidence supports the use of estrogen for stress incontinence, the Mayo Clinic reports that many women find this therapy relieves their urine leakage symptoms.[10] Estrogen is available as a cream, tablets, or a time-release intravaginal ring. Studies indicate that creams are most readily and immediately absorbed by the body, followed by tablets, and then intravaginal rings.[11]

  Side effects: Most women report no side effects of estrogen. Note that estrogen is different from oral hormone replacement, which may worsen incontinence symptoms for some women.

Drugs commonly prescribed for urge urinary incontinence

- **ANTIMUSCARINIC MEDICATION.** This class of drugs is FDA approved for urge incontinence and is effective for alleviating symptoms. See the description of antimuscarinic medication in the previous section on stress urinary incontinence medication. Studies show that this medication is effective in reducing urge incontinence wetting accidents by about two-thirds.[12]
- **TRICYCLIC MEDICATION.** This class of drugs is prescribed for both stress and urge incontinence and has been shown to be effective for both since the drugs relax the bladder and strengthen the internal sphincter to prevent urine leakage.[13] Read more in the description of this class of medications in the previous section on stress urinary incontinence medication.

Drugs commonly prescribed for mixed urinary incontinence

- Your doctor may prescribe medication if you have mixed incontinence, which is usually a combination of stress and urge incontinence. Most women find that their symptoms of one type of incontinence are worse than those of the other, so the more troublesome type is treated first. The medication your doctor prescribes will depend on the type and severity of your symptoms.

Drugs commonly prescribed for decreased sexual sensation

- Although there is little clinical evidence to suggest that estrogen is effective in treating symptoms of decreased sexual sensation, many women report improvement in symptoms with this treatment (especially when used in conjunction with another conservative treatment, like pelvic floor retraining). Studies show that increased estrogen in postmenopausal women is linked with increased sexual satisfaction.[14] Women using this therapy report an increase in vaginal lubrication during sex. See the description of estrogen in the section on medications for treating stress urinary incontinence, earlier in this chapter.

How effective is medication?

Because of the number of available medications to treat urinary incontinence and decreased sexual sensation, as well as the varying levels of symptoms, it is not possible to predict how effective medication will be in treating your condition. When studies have been performed, we offer statistics on the effectiveness of each medication for each condition. By working with your doctor and trying a number of different medications, you can likely find one that will alleviate your symptoms. Most women do not find that medication completely cures their urinary leakage, but most experience a significant reduction in leakage accidents. Many women report improvement in symptoms of decreased sexual sensation with the use of estrogen.

Behavior and Diet Modifications Plus Weight Management

Which conditions does this therapy help?

Many women dealing with one of the three types of urinary incontinence (stress, urge, and mixed), and some who are experiencing pelvic organ prolapse, find that changing lifestyle habits, including managing their weight, can significantly decrease their symptoms. This therapy can also be useful for women who experience decreased sexual sensation.

Who offers this kind of therapy?

Your doctor or therapist can assist you with making lifestyle changes to reduce symptoms of urinary incontinence and pelvic organ prolapse. Therapists who specialize in pelvic floor rehabilitation and urinary incontinence treatment routinely suggest these lifestyle changes.

What do behavior and diet modifications plus weight management involve?

These are three kinds of lifestyle modifications you can make to alleviate urinary incontinence and some symptoms of pelvic organ prolapse:

1. Behavior changes include bladder retraining, stopping smoking, and timing your fluid intake.
2. Diet modifications focus on avoiding foods that irritate your bladder and following a diet that helps you maintain bowel regularity (since constipation strains the pelvic floor muscles, which can worsen your symptoms).
3. If you are overweight, shedding even a few pounds can lessen your symptoms.

Behavior modifications

- BLADDER RETRAINING. Bladder retraining is especially effective for treating urge and mixed incontinence and involves learning to delay urination after you get the urge to go. According to the American Academy of Family Physicians, bladder retraining can help you increase the amount of time between bathroom visits, increase the amount of urine your bladder can hold, and improve your control over the urge to urinate.[15] Most women see results from bladder retraining within three to twelve weeks. To retrain your bladder, use timed voiding, which is the practice of going to the toilet according to the clock rather than waiting for the need to go. You can retrain your bladder using the following steps:
  1. Determine your interval. Before you can set a schedule for timed voiding, you need to first determine how long you can delay urination. At first, attempt to set the interval between bathroom visits at one and a half hours. If you cannot delay for that long, determine what interval works best

for you. The goal of timed voiding is to eventually be able to delay urination for two to three hours.

2. Increase your interval. Once you have determined how long you can currently delay urination, attempt to increase this interval by five to ten minutes. Set a timer to track the interval. If you feel the urge to urinate before your timer goes off, practice any combination of the following techniques to delay urination:
   - Breathe in a controlled and deliberate manner.
   - Visualize a peaceful and tranquil setting.
   - Do a series of quick pelvic floor muscle contractions.
   - Sit quietly and avoid fidgeting.
   - Meditate.
   - Think about something else to distract yourself.

3. Empty your bladder completely. In addition to practicing timed voiding, you can retrain your bladder by ensuring that you empty your bladder completely each time you urinate. After you finish urinating, lean forward and urinate again if necessary. By leaning forward, you change the angle of the bladder neck, which releases any urine left in the bladder.

- STOP SMOKING. Nicotine irritates the bladder, causing urinary urgency and frequency. A smoker's repeated and chronic coughing strains the pelvic floor muscles and may worsen symptoms of stress incontinence. Smoking cessation may help decrease all of these symptoms. Smoking also quadruples the risk of bladder cancer and has the general effect of weakening tissues in the body. Studies reveal that women who smoke are twice as likely to experience symptoms of stress incontinence. Smoking also increases a woman's risk of urinary incontinence in general by 28 percent.[16]

- TIME YOUR FLUID INTAKE. Many women with urinary incontinence operate under the misconception that they need to drastically reduce their fluid intake to alleviate their symptoms, but this is a myth. Too little hydration can worsen urinary incontinence symptoms for two reasons. First, the lack of fluid concentrates the urine, which can irritate the bladder. Second, concentrated urine has a pungent odor, so leakage accidents are more noticeable.[17]

To avoid these problems, you need to drink enough water daily to stay hydrated, usually six to eight cups. If you are at either extreme of the weight scale, drink water in ounces equal to half your body weight (e.g., if you weigh 100 pounds, drink 50 ounces daily). To reduce urinary incontinence symptoms, however, drink most of your water in the morning. Reduce fluid intake after 6 p.m. (or two to three hours before bedtime) to decrease nighttime voiding and incontinence. If still thirsty, use sugar-free candies as needed to keep your mouth moist.

Diet Modifications

- **AVOID BLADDER IRRITANTS.** If you have problems with urinary urgency and frequency, consuming certain foods and beverages can irritate areas of the bladder and urethra that are already inflamed. These foods and drinks tend to make your urine more acidic by decreasing the pH.

  The most common bladder irritants include acidic foods and drinks, caffeine, alcohol, foods containing arylalkylamines (tyrosine, tyramine, tryptophan, aspirate, and phenylalanine), and any foods to which you are allergic. Tables 8.1 and 8.2 list common foods and beverages that are acidic or that contain arylalkylamines. Avoiding these bladder irritants may decrease urge incontinence symptoms. Another option is to supplement meals with an over-the-counter medication like Prelief, which removes acid from foods and drinks.[18] If you are interested in using dietary modification as a way to possibly reduce your symptoms, we suggest that you avoid eating or drinking the items listed in tables 8.1 and 8.2 whenever possible.

  You can replace the fruits listed in table 8.1 with low-acid fruits like apricots, pears, watermelons, and papayas. You can also drink a coffee substitute like Kava or a low-acid instant drink like Postum.

  You may find that your symptoms improve within a few

TABLE 8.1 Acidic foods and beverages to avoid

Alcoholic beverages	Grapes
Apple juice	Guava
Apples	Peaches
Ascorbic acid	Pepper
Cantaloupes	Pineapple
Caffeinated beverages	Plums
Carbonated beverages	Strawberries
Chili peppers, powder, etc.	Tomatoes
Citrus fruits and juices	Vinegar
Cranberries	

weeks after you remove these bladder irritants from your diet. Once your symptoms have improved, you can experiment with adding one food or beverage at a time back into your diet. Notice which ones irritate your bladder and which do not. If you happen to eat or drink something that worsens your symptoms, drink plenty of water to dilute the effect of irritants and reduce urine acidity. You can also increase your water intake when you eat something that irritates your bladder (especially if you just can't resist certain foods).

Bicarbonate slush for emergencies: If your urinary symptoms suddenly become worse, you can try a bicarbonate slush to reduce urine acidity. Simply dilute one tablespoon of baking soda in 16 ounces of water. Drink this slush and immediately drink eight more ounces of water. Consult your doctor before using this slush if you have high blood pressure or are prone to salt retention.[19]

Some people find these dietary changes useful, while others find them too difficult to follow or maintain over a long period. Dietary changes are most effective when combined with other forms of therapy. Regardless, these three methods—avoiding certain foods, increasing your water intake, and using bicarbonate slushes as necessary—do have a positive effect simply by reducing urine acidity.

TABLE 8.2   Arylalkylamine-rich foods and beverages to avoid

Artificial sweeteners	Fava beans	Raisins
Avocados	Lima beans	Rye bread
Bananas	Marmite	Sour cream
Beer	Mayonnaise	Soy sauce
Brewer's yeast	Nuts	Vitamins B and C
Canned figs	Onions	Wine and champagne
Cheese	Pickled herring	Yogurt
Chicken livers	Pineapple	
Chocolate	Prunes	

- MAINTAIN BOWEL REGULARITY. Constipation or straining to have a bowel movement tends to increase pressure on the bladder and can often worsen symptoms of urinary incontinence. To prevent constipation, increase your fiber intake. Eat at least five servings of fruit or vegetables daily. If you still suffer from constipation, an over-the-counter fiber supplement can also help. To mix your own fiber supplement at home, simply combine ¼ cups each of freshly ground flaxseed and aloe vera juice with ½ cup of apple juice. Drink the mixture immediately.[20]

Weight management

- MANAGE YOUR WEIGHT. We can't stress enough the importance of weight management in the treatment of urinary incontinence and pelvic organ prolapse. No therapy, whether conservative or surgical, can ever overcome the forces of obesity. Every single pound of weight from your collarbone down to your pelvic floor pushes down on your bladder. Even small amounts of weight loss can have a dramatic effect.

    One study showed that a 5 to 10 percent loss of weight was as effective as other nonsurgical treatments for incontinence and proposed weight loss as "a first line therapy for incontinence."[21] Another study showed that in an overweight woman, shedding 8 percent of body weight can result in a 47 percent decrease in leakage accidents. Rather than trying to lose weight by yourself, we suggest you join tried-and-true weight loss programs that involve both diet and exercise.

How effective are behavior and diet modifications plus weight management?

Though studies show varying results of lifestyle modification as an effective therapy for urinary incontinence and pelvic organ prolapse, in our practices we see women significantly decrease their symptoms with lifestyle changes. The major benefit of using lifestyle change as a therapy is that, like at-home pelvic floor retraining, you can do it yourself. It empowers you to take action to reduce your symptoms. We see lifestyle changes having the greatest effect most often for women with mild to moderate symptoms who are also trying pelvic floor retraining and medication.

Acupuncture

Which conditions does this therapy help?

Acupuncture is an alternative therapy to treat symptoms of urinary incontinence and pelvic organ prolapse.

Who offers this kind of therapy?

Board-certified acupuncturists as well as doctors offer acupuncture. Check if your doctor or specialist offers this kind of therapy, or ask for a referral for a board-certified acupuncturist if you want to pursue this kind of therapy.

What is acupuncture?

Acupuncture is an ancient Chinese medical practice that is considered an effective alternative therapy for treating symptoms of urine leakage and organ prolapse. An acupuncturist uses very fine needles inserted into the skin at specific points to stimulate and increase the flow of energy in the body. These specific points are located along meridian lines that circulate energy throughout the body, and the use of different combinations of points can create positive healing effects. Acupuncture is well known as a form of pain relief and has been used to treat various conditions, including urinary incontinence. This approach can also alleviate constipation, which in turns relieves pressure in the pelvic region. Depending on your specific condition and the severity of your symptoms, your acupuncturist will design a customized program for you, with the typical treatment period lasting from five to eight weeks.

How effective is acupuncture?

Acupuncture has been shown to help women lessen the severity of symptoms of urinary leakage and prolapse. Researchers Sandra Emmons, M.D., and Lesley Otto, M.D., of Oregon Health and Science University, note that acupuncture is similar in effectiveness to drug therapy or behavior therapy for women with overactive bladder. They add, "Acupuncture perhaps can offer a middle ground for the appropriate patient who prefers not to take a daily medication but is unable to commit to the active involvement of behavioral therapy."[22]

Percutaneous Tibial Nerve Stimulation

Which conditions does this therapy help?

Percutaneous tibial nerve stimulation has been approved within the United States for the treatment of overactive bladder and urge incontinence.[23] This treatment helps women with symptoms of urinary leakage, frequency, and urgency.[24]

Who offers this kind of therapy?

A urologist usually performs percutaneous tibial nerve stimulation, but this treatment can also be delivered by physician assistants and nurses who have received the appropriate training.[25]

What is percutaneous tibial nerve stimulation?

This simple procedure is performed in your doctor's office. As you sit with your leg elevated, a fine needle is inserted into the percutaneous tibial nerve, which is located just above the ankle. A very mild electric current is delivered through the needle to the nerve, which controls bladder function along with other nerves.[26] Your toes or entire foot might flex gently during the treatment, or you might feel a mild tingling sensation in your ankle or in the sole of your foot. The therapy usually involves 30 to 60 minutes of treatment per session, three to four times per week, for 8 to 12 weeks.[27] This conservative treatment is appropriate for patients with overactive bladder or urge incontinence who have not had success with behavior modification or drug therapy.[28] This treatment is also less invasive than sacral neuromodulation, which aims to achieve a similar effect (see chapter 9).

How effective is percutaneous tibial nerve stimulation?

Two studies, the OrBIT trial and the SUMiT trial, demonstrate that percutaneous tibial nerve stimulation is effective for women with overactive bladder who urinate at least eight times every 24 hours.[29] The OrBIT trial showed that women undergoing percutaneous tibial nerve stimulation experienced a 20 percent reduction in frequency of urination. Women in the SUMiT trial experienced about a 36 percent reduction in the severity of their symptoms and more than a 34 percent increase in quality of life.[30] Women undergoing this treatment also reported improvement in urge incontinence, including urinary frequency, urgency, and leakage episodes.[31]

Vaginal Pessaries

Which conditions does this therapy help?

Vaginal pessaries are used mostly to treat pelvic organ prolapse, although they are sometimes used to alleviate symptoms of urinary incontinence.

Who offers this kind of therapy?

Your doctor or your doctor's designated personnel can fit you for a vaginal pessary.

What is a vaginal pessary?

A vaginal pessary is a removable device, usually made of rubber or plastic, inserted into the vagina to support the bladder, uterus, or rectum. Pessaries provide artificial support for pelvic organs that have prolapsed (fallen) out of place. There are several different kinds of pessaries, including rings, cubes, and doughnuts. For a pessary to provide effective relief, it must be appropriate for your condition (type of prolapse) and fit the shape of your vagina. Your gynecologist can fit you with a pessary, with the process requiring one to three office visits. Once a month your pessary needs to be removed and cleaned, either by you or by your physician. Few women experience problems with pessaries, but there is an increased chance of vaginal irritation or infection.

Pessaries are the standard conservative therapy for women with pelvic organ prolapse who wish to avoid surgery, because they either are poor surgical candidates or wish to have more children. Your specialist will choose from the variety of pessaries the type that best suits your type of prolapse and your lifestyle. For instance, supportive pessaries are better for women who are sexually active, while space-occupying pessaries prevent sexual activity but are necessary for women with larger vaginas or women with severe vaginal vault prolapse. Discuss your options carefully with your specialist to find the best pessary for your condition, your body, and your lifestyle.[32]

How effective is a vaginal pessary?

Pessaries are very effective. Studies show that most women with pelvic organ prolapse experience improvement with a pessary, and for some women symptoms go away completely.[33] Well-fitted pessaries relieve prolapse symptoms for 70 to 90 percent of women, while an additional 40 to 60 percent of women experience an improvement in sexual activity. Vaginal pessaries also successfully treat 40 to 50 percent of women who have urinary incontinence symptoms as a result of their pelvic organ prolapse.[34]

Urethral Dilation

Very rarely, a narrowing of the urethral opening, called a urethral stricture, can cause symptoms of urge incontinence or overactive bladder. Despite the lack of evidence to support urethral dilation as an effective treatment for these symptoms, gentle urethral dilation has been anecdotally reported to benefit a small number of women.[35] We include urethral dilation in this chapter for historical perspective. This treatment option was much more popular decades ago, and women occasionally still request urethral dilation from their urologists. For some women this is a one-time procedure. Other women benefit from having urethral dilation periodically, from every six months to every two years. Some controversy surrounds this treatment option since it is effective for only a limited number of women and, to date, no evidence-based research proves its efficacy for overactive bladder or urge incontinence.

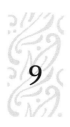

9

Surgical Solutions

When conservative treatments are not effective, women who have severe or especially uncomfortable urinary incontinence or pelvic organ prolapse may require surgery. There are many surgical procedures to correct the situation, including more than one hundred surgeries to correct stress urinary incontinence alone. The more common procedures are primarily intended to correct pelvic organ prolapse and urinary incontinence caused by prolapse, including stress urinary incontinence, overactive bladder, urge urinary incontinence, or mixed urinary incontinence (see table 9.1 for the success rates of the most common procedures). Surgeries to correct pelvic floor conditions fall into five major categories:

1. Transobturator tape and tension-free vaginal tape procedures to address stress urinary incontinence
   • Transobturator tape
   • Single-incision transobturator tape
   • Tension-free vaginal tape
2. Pubovaginal sling procedures to address stress urinary incontinence
3. Open procedures to address stress urinary incontinence
   • Burch procedure
   • Marshall-Marchetti-Krantz procedure

4. Procedures to address pelvic organ prolapse
   - Cystocele repair
   - Rectocele repair
   - Enterocele repair
   - Vaginal vault repair, or sacral colpopexy
   - Uterine suspension procedures
   - Hysterectomy
5. Sacral neuromodulation to address overactive bladder, urge urinary incontinence, urge-dominant mixed urinary incontinence, and urinary retention

General Principles and Precautions with Transvaginal Surgery

With any transvaginal surgery, depending on the extent of the repair being performed, your physician may use either general anesthesia or regional (spinal) or local anesthesia with sedation. You may need to stay in the hospital overnight. A small percentage of patients may experience complications, generally associated with any surgery, from the procedures discussed in this chapter.

Risks of any surgical procedure

Although most of the surgical procedures we discuss in this chapter are minimally invasive, with some taking just 10 minutes for the actual procedure, all surgeries have inherent risks. You doctor should discuss the general risks of any surgery with you, as well as any specific risks associated with any medical conditions you might have. According to the National Institutes of Health, the risks for any surgery include:[1]

- Infection at the site of the incision(s)
- Incision(s) opening up
- Blood clots in the legs that may move to the lungs
- Bleeding
- Other infection

TABLE 9.1 Surgical procedure success rates

Surgical procedure	Used to treat	Invasiveness	Success rates
Transobturator tape	Stress urinary incontinence	Minimal	85%–95%
Single-incision transobturator tape	Stress urinary incontinence	Minimal	66%–90%
Tension-free vaginal tape	Stress urinary incontinence	Minimal	81%
Pubovaginal sling	Stress urinary incontinence	Moderate	81% with synthetic mesh 70%–95% with tissue
Burch procedure	Stress urinary incontinence	Moderate	Above 80% (especially with laparoscopic approach)
Marshall-Marchetti-Krantz procedure	Stress urinary incontinence	Moderate	71% short term 28%–57% long term
Cystocele repair	Cystocele (bladder hernia)	Moderate	80%–93% without mesh augmentation 89%–92% with mesh augmentation
Rectocele repair	Rectocele (large intestine hernia)	Moderate	93% with graft augmentation 24% improvement in sexual satisfaction
Enterocele repair	Enterocele (small intestine hernia)	Moderate	82%–96%
Sacral colpopexy	Vaginal vault prolapse	Moderate	81%–97%
Sacral neuromodulation	Overactive bladder, urge urinary incontinence, urge-dominant mixed urinary incontinence, urinary retention	Minimal	31%–65%

Postoperative guidelines

To reduce the chance of complications, be sure to follow your physician's postoperative guidelines. These general guidelines will give you an idea of what to expect:[2]

1. Call your physician immediately if you develop a fever above 101 degrees, extreme chills, or severe pain that is not alleviated by pain medication.
2. Do not use tampons or engage in sexual activity for six weeks.
3. Do not drive for 48 hours after surgery. If you are not taking narcotic pain pills, you may drive after two days.
4. For up to a month after surgery, you might experience some vaginal spotting.
5. You may shower after surgery, but avoid tub baths, swimming, and hot tubs for two weeks.
6. Avoid vigorous physical activity immediately after surgery, and do not lift more than 10 pounds for six weeks. You may walk as much as desired and go up and down stairs.
7. Do not strain to have bowel movements. Be aware that pain medications can sometimes cause constipation. To avoid constipation, use a stool softener or milk of magnesia as often as needed. You can also make and drink a homemade mixture for constipation relief: grind ¼ cup of flaxseed and mix it with ½ cup of apple juice and ¼ cup of aloe vera juice. Be sure to grind the flaxseed fresh each time and drink the mixture immediately.
8. You may experience urinary leakage on your way to the bathroom. This is a normal symptom and usually stops as your body heals.
9. There are usually no diet restrictions after surgery.
10. With the exception of blood thinners, you may resume your daily medications or hormones as soon as you are released

from the hospital. Consult your physician about taking blood thinners after surgery.

Of course, if you have any complications or postoperative questions or concerns, don't be afraid to talk to your physician. Remember that you, as the patient, are at the core of a patient-centered care model. You had enough courage to talk to your physician about urinary incontinence or pelvic organ prolapse in the first place. Don't let that courage fail you here. Ask questions and express any concerns to your physician, because peace of mind is sometimes the best medicine for healing.

General Considerations for Incontinence Surgeries

All surgeries for incontinence carry their own risks, some greater than others. In this section we cover the general risks to consider when contemplating incontinence surgery, which include surgeries to correct stress incontinence, overactive bladder or urge incontinence, and urge-dominant mixed urinary incontinence.

Both the transobturator tape and tension-free vaginal tape procedures are minimally invasive and often require lower levels of anesthesia than other incontinence surgeries. The risks associated with these surgeries are low, similar to those of other vaginal procedures. In addition to the general risks associated with any surgery, risks associated with these procedures include:[3]

- Temporary urinary retention (requiring the use of a catheter for up to six weeks)
- Permanent urinary retention (due to overtightening of the tape, requiring additional surgery to correct)
- Onset of urge incontinence or overactive bladder, including irritable bladder
- Recurrent stress incontinence due to mesh or sling failure
- Sling erosion into pelvic organs when synthetic sling materials are used

- Recurrent urinary tract infections
- Groin pain (occurs rarely)

Pubovaginal sling procedures carry the additional risk of bladder perforation, as is true with all procedures that require surgeons to use needles near the bladder. Bladder perforation can cause significant complications. If the surgeon realizes the bladder is perforated at the time of surgery, the patient will need to wear a catheter for seven to ten days. If bladder perforation is not recognized at the time of surgery, the patient can leak urine into the pelvis and can develop an abnormal connection between the bladder and the vagina. Surgeons not experienced in operating in retropubic space—the region between the pubic symphysis (a joint located directly above a woman's genitalia) and the bladder—increase the risk of bladder perforation. Because of this risk, fewer pubovaginal sling procedures were performed in 2010. With this kind of procedure, tissue degradation is also a risk when tissue grafts are used.[4]

Open procedures for incontinence, such as the Burch and Marshall-Marchetti-Krantz procedures, also present additional risks, including the formation of fistulas (abnormal connections between pelvic organs) and larger than normal incisions for laparoscopic procedures if complications occur.[5]

Transobturator Tape

What is a transobturator tape procedure?

The transobturator tape is a minimally invasive procedure designed to prevent stress incontinence by supporting the urethra and holding it in place. As you probably recall from the anatomy discussion in chapter 1, the urethra is the tube that allows urine to flow out of the bladder, and it is normally supported by strong pelvic ligaments. When these ligaments become dislodged or weakened, for any number of reasons, the result can be hypermobility of the urethra. This means that the urethra is no longer held in place, which can cause urinary leakage, specifically stress incontinence and intrinsic sphincter dysfunction.

Who are ideal candidates for this surgery?

This procedure is an ideal surgical solution for women with pure stress urinary incontinence who have limited vaginal access. Limited vaginal access means a narrow vagina. Women can have a narrow vagina due to age, radiation treatment, lack of estrogen, and having never delivered vaginally. The transobturator tape is an especially good option for women with stress incontinence who have had trouble staying dry using conservative approaches. This procedure can also work well for prolapse patients and can be done with other prolapse repairs, such as enterocele or cystocele repair, uterine suspension, or hysterectomy.

How does this surgery work?

There are two forms of transobturator tape procedures: one that requires three incisions and one that requires a single incision. With both procedures, a piece of mesh or tape is surgically placed around the urethra to provide support. The tape exerts no tension on the urethra. It merely provides stability during episodes of increased intra-abdominal pressure that would result in urine leakage, such as when you cough, lift, or strain. The tape or mesh is permanent, and your body's healing response anchors it in place. As a result, the urethra becomes stable, and urine leakage is reduced or eliminated. This procedure is currently being performed on women ages 20 to 90.

How invasive is this surgery?

The transobturator tape procedure is minimally invasive and can be performed alone or in conjunction with other pelvic prolapse procedures. The surgeon may opt for sedation plus local anesthesia, regional (or spinal) anesthesia, or general anesthesia, depending on the medical condition and age of the patient, as well as whether other procedures will be performed at the same time.

If performed alone, transobturator tape is usually done as an outpatient procedure. Most women go home the same day. One factor that makes this surgery minimally invasive is that the actual procedure takes only 10 to 20 minutes. With this surgery, patients experience little intra-operative bladder injury, decreased convalescence time and blood loss, and less urinary retention compared with most other procedures to correct incontinence.[6] There is also less risk that the patient's bowel or blood vessels will be injured.[7]

The single-incision procedure is even less invasive than the procedure requiring three incisions and has the following additional benefits:

- Decreased anesthetic requirement
- Less pain after surgery
- Often shorter recovery period than after the triple-incision procedure
- Reduced risk of injury to surrounding organs, such as bladder and bowels[8]

How is this surgery performed?

The triple-incision procedure requires a small vaginal incision and two very small incisions on either side of the vaginal opening. A piece of mesh or tape is passed through a hole in the pelvic bone called the obturator fossa. The obturator fossa houses the obturator nerve and vessels. Multiple types of synthetic mesh and tape are available, and most have about the same success rates. Special curved needles are used to place the tape or mesh. It is not attached to pelvic bone, ligaments, or muscles but is instead permanently anchored into place by the body's own healing process.

With the single-incision surgery, an incision is made in the anterior vagina (the side closest to the urethra), and a specially designed piece of mesh tape is passed into the obturator internus muscle on either side of the urethra, near its middle. A single incision means the tape has nowhere to exit. Instead, the tape used in this procedure has points on either end that anchor in the obturator internus muscle. As your body heals, tissues (called fibroblasts) grow into the mesh, holding the tape permanently in place. Many surgeons prefer this procedure over the regular approach because some studies show that tape placement is more accurate and that bladder injury is less likely.[9]

Most patients can urinate before they leave the hospital, and occasionally, the patient must go home with a catheter for one night. If you go home with a catheter, you should call your doctor's office to have it removed the next day.

What are the success rates for this surgery?

The triple-incision procedure is very effective for women with pure stress urinary incontinence. According to research, women who undergo transobturator tape surgery have a success rate ranging from 85 to 95 percent in terms of symptom improvement or staying completely dry.[10] The single-incision surgery also has a high success rate, around 85 to 90 percent, with a 66 percent success rate after one year.[11] Success rates decrease over time due to many factors: gravity, weight gain, or chronic cough, for example. Triple-incision rates are about the same.

Tension-Free Vaginal Tape

What is a tension-free vaginal tape procedure?

Tension-free vaginal tape is designed to prevent urine leakage from stress incontinence. As with the transobturator tape surgery, the goal of this procedure is to support and stabilize a urethra that is hypermobile because of weakened pelvic floor muscles or ligaments. If you have stress urinary incontinence, tension-free vaginal tape will stabilize both the bladder neck and the urethra when you cough or sneeze, as well as keeping the urethral seal tight and preventing urine from leaving the bladder. Tension-free vaginal tape material may be synthetic mesh, tissue from the patient, or tissue from a cadaver.

This procedure has also been used in attempts to cure urge and mixed incontinence, although the results are mixed at best.[12] Most surgeons opt for this approach only for women who have pure stress urinary incontinence. The National Institute for Clinical Excellence, after appraising the tension-free vaginal tape procedure, has "recommended tension-free vaginal tape as one option for the surgical treatment of women with stress incontinence whenever non-surgical treatments (such as pelvic floor exercises) have not worked."[13]

Who are ideal candidates for this surgery?

This procedure is ideal for women with stress incontinence who have not had success with less invasive surgical procedures or who have had multiple failed incontinence surgeries. Tension-free vaginal tape also appears to be a safe and effective method for obese women seeking relief from stress urinary incontinence.[14]

How does this surgery work?

Tension-free vaginal tape is designed to support the urethra and bladder neck like a hammock whenever intra-abdominal pressure increases, such as when you exercise or lift a heavy object. The theory behind transobturator tape and tension-free vaginal tape procedures are similar. But the method of placement and the durability of tension-free vaginal tape make it a more suitable solution for the group of women described as ideal candidates: those who have had failed incontinence surgeries, obese women, or women with severe incontinence.

How invasive is this surgery?

Unlike transobturator tape procedures, which are minimally invasive, the tension-free vaginal tape procedure is considered moderately invasive because of the way the tape is inserted in the body. Depending on the surgical approach, there is the added risk that the tape may exert too much tension on the urethra, causing difficulty with postoperative urination. Although this problem doesn't happen often, when it does occur, the surgeon needs to perform a short secondary surgery to loosen the tape. Within 5 to 10 days after the procedure, the surgeon can loosen the tape through the vaginal incision.

But if the tape is not adjusted within this time frame, the patient will need to use a catheter to help with urination for four weeks, or until the body has healed and the mesh is fixed into position. After that, the surgeon can release tension on the tape by a different method.

Tension-free vaginal tape surgery is considered even more invasive if the surgeon uses your own (autologous) tissue, because this requires additional incisions to harvest the tissue.

How is this surgery performed?

In tension-free vaginal tape surgery, a long needle is used to pass tissue or mesh from the vagina to the suprapubic space (the area above the pubic arch), or vice versa. This long piece of material can be attached in various ways. Like the transobturator tape, the tension-free vaginal tape supports the urethra. Unlike the transobturator tape, the tension-free vaginal tape is not placed around the urethra via the hole in the pelvic bone (called the obturator fossa). Instead, the route of insertion is more "vertical" and the material is further from the surface of the skin.

One unique aspect of the tension-free vaginal tape procedure is that your surgeon will probably ask you to cough during or just after the procedure. This allows him or her to check the tension on the mesh tape, ensuring that it is not placed too tightly. Studies show that proper adjustment of the tape both cures urinary incontinence symptoms and prevents voiding difficulties after the surgery.[15] Many surgeons will choose to use sedation and local anesthesia for this procedure because they allow you to be awake for the cough test. Other surgeons opt to use manual lower-abdominal wall pressure to simulate the cough test, especially if general anesthesia is used. Studies show that both approaches are equally effective.[16] Regional (spinal) anesthesia plus sedation has also been used.

Once the tension-free vaginal tape is placed, it can be anchored to the body in various ways, including tying sutures to the pelvic fascia (a band or sheet of strong fibrous connective tissue), anchoring the tape to the pubic bone, or tying sutures to each other over the fascia. Your surgeon will choose the procedure that best suits your incontinence needs.

Be aware that multiple kinds of synthetic mesh tape or your own or donor tissue can be used for this procedure. If you are considering this type of surgery to alleviate your stress incontinence symptoms, you may wish to ask your surgeon about the type of tape that would best fit your health situation. Currently, surgeons favor a loosely knitted polypropylene mesh because this material has the correct amount of elasticity to support the urethra without being too stiff, which can lead to mesh erosion. The loosely woven mesh also allows infection-fighting cells to enter the surgery site, decreasing the risk of infection. Many surgeons opt for synthetic materials for the mesh especially when the patient has already had a failed surgery at the same site.[17]

What are the success rates for this surgery?

The tension-free vaginal tape procedure has a success rate of 81 percent after about seven and a half years.[18] The surgery improves or cures urinary incontinence,[19] with low rates of mesh erosion over time.[20] A positive aspect of the tension-free vaginal tape procedure is that the relatively high success rates are stable over time, meaning that a woman who has her urinary incontinence cured by this surgery is likely to stay cured.[21]

Pubovaginal Sling Procedures

What is a pubovaginal sling procedure?

The pubovaginal sling is primarily used to treat stress urinary incontinence of all degrees of severity. In the procedure, a piece of material is placed either mid-urethra or directly under the bladder neck (proximal urethra). The goal of the sling is to stabilize and support the bladder neck and urethra when there is intra-abdominal stress, such as when you exercise, cough, or pick up a heavy object. This surgery may also increase the pressure and effectiveness of the urethral seal, which can prevent urine leakage caused by stress incontinence.

Several types of pubovaginal sling surgeries were used in the past to address stress incontinence—the Stamey, Raz, and Gittes procedures. These surgeries also used long needles and sutures to anchor the bladder neck or urethra to pelvic fibrous tissues or to the pubic bone. These procedures are now rarely used, however, since they have higher associated failure rates and risks compared with modern pubovaginal sling methods.

Who are ideal candidates for this surgery?

The pubovaginal sling is ideal for women who have had failed stress incontinence surgeries as well as women who are undergoing prolapse procedures when there is a potential for postsurgical incontinence. In addition, women who are prone to high intra-abdominal pressure make ideal candidates for this sling. This includes obese women, in whom excess weight puts a lot of downward pressure on the pelvic floor, as well as athletes and women who suffer from a persistent cough, such as those with chronic pulmonary disease.

How does this surgery work?

As the name implies, the pubovaginal sling procedure involves passing a piece of sling material from the suprapubic space (the area above the pubic bone), through the tissues anterior to (in front of) the vagina, around the mid-urethra or directly under the bladder neck, and then back up into the suprapubic space on the other side of the midline. The sling acts like a hammock, preventing the urethra and bladder neck from descending (called urethral hypermobility) when intra-abdominal pressure increases, keeping urine in the bladder, and preventing leakage. The sling can also support the urethral seal, which can help when the urethra's closing pressure is not enough to keep urine in the bladder under stress (a condition called an intrinsic sphincter deficiency, or ISD).

How invasive is this surgery?

Like the tension-free vaginal tape procedure, the pubovaginal sling approach is moderately invasive for several reasons. First, if the surgeon is using your tissue (autologous tissue) to create the sling, this means at least one extra incision during surgery. Second, the surgeon often uses long thin needles to pass the sling through the body, so there is some risk of damage to the bladder. Because this is a moderately invasive procedure, most surgeons elect to use general anesthesia, although regional (spinal) anesthesia with sedation is also sometimes used.

How is this surgery performed?

Incisions will be made in the vagina and the abdomen. Some versions of this procedure also require incisions in the thigh. To place the pubovaginal sling, the surgeon places a length of sling material mid-urethra or directly under the bladder neck, usually using long thin needles. The surgeon may choose to use your tissue, donor tissue from a cadaver (human or porcine), or a synthetic material, like polypropylene mesh, for the sling. As with the tension-free vaginal tape procedure, it is best to talk with your surgeon about which material best suits your situation.

The surgeon may attach the sling by tying the sutures to the fascia (connective tissue) in the suprapubic space, by using bone anchors to connect the sling to the pubic bone, or by tying sutures to each other over the fascia.

What are the success rates for this surgery?

The pubovaginal sling has relatively high rates of cure for women with stress urinary incontinence. Eighty-one percent of women who had a synthetic pubovaginal sling were completely continent at 24 months, and an additional 16 percent showed improvement with mild stress incontinence.[22] Slings created with donor or autologous tissue have reported initial success rates of 70 to 95 percent,[23] but they have a higher risk of degrading over time. Because of this, many surgeons are now using synthetic mesh, despite the higher risks of mesh erosion and infection.

Burch Procedure

What is the Burch procedure, or Burch colposuspension?

The Burch procedure is one of more than one hundred surgical procedures that have been performed since 1910 to correct stress incontinence and is one of the oldest procedures with long-term success rates. The Burch procedure is a modification of the Marshall-Marchetti-Krantz procedure (another open procedure, described later in this chapter). As with most surgeries designed to correct stress incontinence, the goal of this procedure is to prevent urethral hypermobility, when the urethra and bladder neck descend as abdominal pressure increases. This surgery also aims to increase resting urethral closing pressure. When closing pressure isn't enough (called intrinsic sphincter deficiency), urine can leak from the bladder. This deficiency is another cause of stress urinary incontinence. The Burch procedure is also called a bladder neck suspension or a Burch colposuspension.

Who are ideal candidates for this surgery?

Because the Burch procedure is more invasive when done as an open surgery, and requires more skilled surgery when done as a laparoscopic procedure, it is currently recommended primarily for women who can't have a synthetic sling or who wish to have children in the future.[24]

How does this surgery work?

The Burch procedure works like the tension-free vaginal tape and other sling procedures except it uses direct suturing rather than a piece of tape to reposition the urethra and bladder neck. The Burch procedure relies on sutures and the strength of the patient's own pelvic tissue, bone, and ligaments to support the bladder.

How invasive is this surgery?

The Burch procedure is moderately invasive, taking from one to two hours to complete. General anesthesia is used when this procedure is done abdominally, and either general or spinal (regional) anesthesia plus sedation can be used when this procedure is performed laparoscopically. Your surgeon will decide the best approach based on your age and general medical condition. As with other moderately invasive incontinence surgeries, you might need to stay in the hospital for one to two days after the procedure, and you might go home with a catheter.

How is this surgery performed?

There are three approaches to performing the Burch procedure: open abdominal, laparoscopic, and transvaginal. In the open abdominal procedure, an incision about three to five inches long is made in the lower abdomen. The bladder is located through the incision, along with the urethra and vagina. The surgeon inserts a finger in the vagina to help locate the position for sutures, then places sutures on either side of the urethra, the bladder neck, and the vaginal wall. After repositioning and lifting these organs, the surgeon then attaches these sutures directly to the pelvic bones or ligaments (usually Cooper's ligament) to secure the position of these organs.

In the laparoscopic procedure, the surgeon makes smaller incisions (about an inch long) in the abdomen, which makes this approach less invasive. The third approach, the transvaginal procedure, is also considered less invasive and achieves the same repositioning of the bladder and urethra through incisions in the vagina.

What are the success rates for this surgery?

The Burch procedure has been performed over a longer period than most other retropubic suspension procedures. Published studies report that the procedure shows relatively high success rates, of 69 to

100 percent, with most rates above 80 percent, especially for the laparoscopic approach.[25] In addition, studies show that when the Burch procedure is done at the same time as a sacral colpopexy to prevent stress urinary incontinence caused by pelvic organ prolapse, patients have significantly reduced stress incontinence symptoms.[26] Some surgeons still consider the Burch procedure to be the gold standard for surgeries to correct stress incontinence because of its long-term success rates.

Marshall-Marchetti-Krantz Procedure

What is the Marshall-Marchetti-Krantz procedure?

Like the Burch procedure, the Marshall-Marchetti-Krantz procedure is designed to alleviate stress incontinence symptoms. This surgery is also called a bladder neck suspension or a vesicourethropexy. Similar to other stress urinary incontinence surgeries, this procedure raises and repositions the urethra and the bladder neck. This decreases urethral hypermobility (prevents the bladder neck and urethra from descending when abdominal pressure increases), preventing urine leakage.

Who are ideal candidates for this surgery?

Because other surgeries for stress urinary incontinence have high success rates, the Marshall-Marchetti-Krantz procedure is not often used. This approach is recommended for women who have not had previous incontinence surgeries.

How does this surgery work?

The Marshall-Marchetti-Krantz procedure, like the Burch procedure, relies on sutures and the strength of the patient's own pelvic tissues and ligaments to hold the repositioned urethra and bladder neck. (Compare with other procedures, such as the pubovaginal sling, which combines sutures with a mesh that supports the urethra like a hammock.)

How invasive is this surgery?

This procedure, like the Burch, is moderately invasive and can require up to two hours to complete. When this procedure is performed abdominally, general anesthesia is used. A laparoscopic approach calls for either general or spinal (regional) anesthesia plus sedation. Your surgeon will help you decide which approach best suits your medical needs. Expect to stay in the hospital for a day or two after this procedure because it is moderately invasive. You may also need to go home with a catheter.

How is this surgery performed?

The Marshall-Marchetti-Krantz procedure can be performed as either an open abdominal surgery or a laparoscopic surgery. With the open abdominal approach, an incision is made in the lower abdomen, and the bladder and other pelvic organs are identified. The surgeon inserts a finger in the vagina to identify the location for suture placement. Sutures are placed in tissues near the bladder neck and urethra, or in the anterior bladder wall. The surgeon then lifts the urethra or the bladder (or both), and secures it in this raised position by attaching the sutures to the pubic bone or to the tissues (fascia) above the pubic bone. These sutures help hold the upper part of the urethra and the bladder in the raised position, preventing stress incontinence symptoms. The lack of hammock support from below lowers the success rate of this procedure compared with transvaginal slings or tapes. The laparoscopic procedure is similar but requires smaller incisions.

What are the success rates for this surgery?

One reason this procedure is not used as often as other stress urinary incontinence surgeries is that it has a lower success rate. Women who have had this procedure report short- or medium-term relief from stress incontinence symptoms, but symptoms seem to recur over the long term. For instance, 43 percent of women who had the Marshall-Marchetti-Krantz surgery had recurrent incontinence symptoms after five years, and 72 percent showed symptoms after a decade.[27] Success rates are higher when patients do not have pelvic organ prolapse and when the bladder is stable prior to surgery.[28]

General Considerations for Pelvic Organ Prolapse Surgeries

Risks of procedures that address pelvic organ prolapse

Possible but rare complications related to surgical procedures that address pelvic organ prolapse include:[29]

- Bladder perforation and rectal injury
- Urinary incontinence
- Temporary and permanent urinary retention
- Mild temporary buttock pain
- Pelvic pain or painful postsurgical sexual intercourse
- Formation of fistulas (abnormal connections between organs)
- Mesh erosion or infection (if synthetic materials are involved)
- Degradation of graft tissue (if graft tissue is used)
- Vaginal foreshortening or narrowing of the vaginal wall
- Heavy bleeding

Cystocele Repair

What is cystocele repair?

This surgical procedure corrects a cystocele, which is a hernia of the bladder. With a cystocele, the structures supporting the bladder weaken, and the bladder descends into the vagina. Women with cystoceles may or may not have urinary incontinence. Occasionally some women with very large cystoceles may have trouble emptying the bladder.

Who are ideal candidates for this surgery?

Cystocele repair is done on women with diagnosed cystoceles and may be performed with other prolapse or urinary incontinence procedures. This surgery is ideal for women who currently show symptoms of their cystocele, including urinary incontinence, urinary obstruction (which can lead to recurrent urinary tract infections), discomfort from the prolapse, or painful sexual intercourse.

How does this surgery work?

The goal of cystocele repair is to reposition the bladder, as much as possible, in its correct anatomical place using sutures. If the cystocele is large, the surgeon might elevate the bladder using a synthetic piece of mesh. Cystocele repair is done through incisions in the vagina.

How invasive is this surgery?

The cystocele repair procedure is moderately invasive because of the length of the surgery and the type of anesthesia used. General anesthesia is most frequently used for this surgery, although some surgeons perform this procedure as an outpatient surgery, depending on the age and general medical condition of the patient. Some patients might require a one- to two-day hospital stay and might need to use a catheter for a period after the surgery.

How is this surgery performed?

With a normal cystocele repair, the surgeon makes an incision in the anterior (front) vaginal wall and identifies the tissues that have separated to allow the cystocele to occur. The weakened bladder is repositioned using sutures to strengthen the weakened pelvic fascia (tissue), which normally holds the bladder in place. Because a chronic bladder protrusion can cause excess vaginal wall tissue to develop, the surgeon may need to remove the excess tissue before closing the incision with sutures. This entire procedure is called an anterior colporrhaphy.

If the cystocele is large or recurring, the surgeon might also perform a cystocele repair augmentation. This procedure involves elevating and supporting the bladder with a piece of synthetic mesh (although biological grafts have been used in the past).

What are the success rates for this surgery?

Straightforward cystocele repairs have relatively high success rates, around 93 percent after 13 months,[30] although some studies show poorer outcomes, with as much as 20 percent of women having recurrent prolapses.[31] The more complex cystocele surgeries, which include augmentation with synthetic mesh, have success rates of 89 to 92 percent in a 6- to 34-month period.[32]

Rectocele Repair

What is rectocele repair?

Similar to cystocele repair, rectocele repair also corrects a prolapse. A rectocele is a herniation of the large intestine, or rectum, which pushes against the posterior (back) wall of the vagina. This herniation can create a pocket just above the anal sphincter in which stool can become trapped. Since a rectocele is a weakness in the tissues supporting the rectum rather than a defect of the rectum, rectocele surgery repairs the supporting structures rather than rectal tissue.

Who are ideal candidates for this surgery?

Surgery to correct a rectocele is recommended for patients experiencing symptoms such as protrusion of the hernia into the entrance of the vagina, physical discomfort, unsatisfying sex, chronic constipation, incomplete defecation, urinary incontinence, or difficulty with urination. If surgery is delayed, a woman may experience painful vaginal wall ulceration from the rectocele. This surgery is not recommended for women who still want to have children.

How does this surgery work?

The goal of rectocele repair is to restore the correct position and function of the vagina while strengthening the vaginal wall tissues to prevent recurrent relapse. In doing so, the repair, which may or may not be augmented with mesh, is intended to alleviate the symptoms associated with the rectocele. Additional surgical procedures, such as enterocele repair, cystocele repair, other urinary incontinence repair procedures, or hysterectomy may be done at the same time.

How invasive is this surgery?

Rectocele repair has the same moderate level of invasiveness as cystocele repair. Because of the length of the surgery and the possible need to perform additional surgical procedures at the same time, surgeons generally perform this repair with the patient under general anesthesia, although some surgeons choose regional (spinal) anesthesia with sedation for simpler versions of this procedure. Many patients require a short hospital stay of one to two days. The medical condition and age of the patient often dictate the type of anesthesia, surgical approach, and recovery plan.

How is this surgery performed?

Before undergoing a rectocele repair, the patient is generally given an enema as well as preoperative antibiotics to prevent infection. In the procedure, the surgeon makes an incision in the posterior (back) vaginal wall. This incision extends all the way down to the perineum (the area between the anus and the vagina, or the opening to the vagina, including the internal associated muscular structures). Once the incision is made, the rectum is identified and pushed back into place. The surgeon then reinforces and strengthens the fascia (tissue) between the rectum and the vagina using sutures alone or a combination of sutures and mesh. For the mesh, surgeons may choose to use your (autologous) tissue, donor tissue (human cadaver or porcine), or a synthetic material.

If excess vaginal tissue has developed because the vagina has been overstretched or because the rectocele has been chronic, the surgeon may remove the excess tissue. If additional surgical procedures are to be performed, these are usually completed before the rectocele repair.

Additional surgical procedures can be done at the junction of the vaginal vault (the top end of the vagina) and the perineum to tighten the vaginal opening. This can restore or increase the pleasure of sexual intercourse for both a woman and her partner. The surgeon also makes sure that the vaginal opening will be large enough, after the surgery, for the patient to experience pain-free intercourse.

What are the success rates for this surgery?

Rectocele repair appears to be highly successful. Recurrence of rectoceles is "extremely uncommon,"[33] which is untrue of other types of prolapse. One study conducted with Brigham and Women's Hospital of Harvard University demonstrated that graft-augmented techniques had a 93 percent success rate.[34] In another study, 90 percent of patients reported improvement in previously difficult bowel evacuation.[35] The results for sexual satisfaction are mixed. One study showed that 24 percent of women who'd had rectocele repair reported improvement in their sexual satisfaction postsurgery, but 9 percent reported deterioration in satisfaction.[36] Success rates overall appear to be higher if a patient can avoid constipation postsurgery and does not become pregnant and deliver vaginally.[37]

Enterocele Repair

What is enterocele repair?

Enterocele repair corrects a hernia of the small bowel, or small intestine. An enterocele occurs when the small bowel presses against and moves into the upper wall of the vagina, causing the vaginal wall to bulge. Enteroceles often occur after surgical procedures that change the angle of the vagina, especially hysterectomies. They are commonly found in conjunction with cystoceles, rectoceles, and uterine prolapse.

Who are ideal candidates for this surgery?

Surgery to repair an enterocele is performed on women with diagnosed enteroceles, which may not become symptomatic until they become so large that they bulge significantly into the vagina. Symptoms include a pulling sensation in the pelvic region or low-back pain, both of which are improved when the patient lies down. Enterocele repairs are also recommended when a pessary is ineffective, often because the patient has difficulty placing or removing the pessary or because the pessary is a physically poor fit. Enterocele repair is not recommended for women who experience relief with a pessary, are high-risk surgical candidates, have minimal symptoms, or want to have children in the future.

How does this surgery work?

As with the cystocele and rectocele repair surgeries, the goal of enterocele repair is to reposition the prolapsed organ and close the gap caused by the weakened pelvic tissue. The defect is in the vaginal tissue rather than in the intestinal tissue. This procedure is usually performed through the vagina rather than through the abdomen.

How invasive is this surgery?

Enterocele repair is moderately invasive for several reasons. First, the procedure is often performed at the same time as other pelvic organ repairs. Second, the length of the surgery is about the same as that of cystocele and rectocele procedures, which is longer than simpler procedures like the transobturator tape or tension-free vaginal tape. Finally, depending on the patient's medical condition, age, and health risks, the surgeon might opt for general anesthesia rather than regional (spinal) anesthesia with sedation. Some patients will need to use a catheter for a few days and might need to recuperate in the hospital for one to two days after the surgery.

How is this surgery performed?

To repair the enterocele, an incision is made near the upper end of the vagina, where the prolapse has occurred. Once the enterocele (prolapsed sac) is identified through the incisions, it is gently teased free from the surrounding tissues. Then an incision is made in the peritoneum, which is a large membrane in the abdominal cavity that supports the internal organs. The prolapsed sac is pushed back into the abdomen, the excess peritoneum tissue is removed, and the incision is closed. If excess vaginal tissue has developed because the prolapse was chronic, this excess tissue will be removed before the vaginal incision is also closed.

Similar to the cystocele and rectocele repairs, the surgeon might choose to augment the repair with synthetic mesh or a tissue graft if necessary. Mesh material is synthetic, and graft material may come from donor tissue (human or porcine) or autologous tissue (your own).

What are the success rates for this surgery?

The success rate of enterocele repair is difficult to pinpoint since experts do not even agree on the definition of an enterocele. In addition, because enteroceles are often asymptomatic, women with this condition are often not even aware that they have a prolapse, or they are more bothered by other types of prolapse.[38] Studies that show definite results report an 82 percent cure rate for patients who undergo simple enterocele repair, and a 96 percent cure rate in patients who also had vaginal vault prolapse.[39] Generally, women who had surgery at the same time for both pelvic organ prolapse and enterocele reported an improvement in their prolapse symptoms.[40] Enteroceles are reported to recur in about 10 percent of women postsurgery.[41]

Vaginal Vault Repair, or Sacral Colpopexy

What is sacral colpopexy?

Sacral colpopexy is designed to repair vaginal vault prolapse, in which the upper part of the vagina sags, often dropping down into the vagina or even outside the vagina. A vault prolapse often occurs because the supporting tissues around and above the vagina slip down. This kind of prolapse can occur at the same time as cystoceles, rectoceles, and enteroceles. Weaknesses in the vaginal and pelvic tissues and muscles contribute to vaginal vault prolapse.

Who are ideal candidates for this surgery?

Women who have vaginal vault prolapse with moderate to severe symptoms that cannot be resolved with conservative measures like pessaries are ideal candidates for sacral colpopexy. Symptoms include incontinence, bulging tissue in the vagina (causing difficulty walking, standing, or with sexual intercourse), a heavy feeling in the pelvis, low-back pain, or vaginal bleeding.

How does this surgery work?

A sacral colpopexy procedure can be approached several ways. In general, the surgery restores the appropriate length of the vagina after it has prolapsed, or fallen, by attaching the apex (top) of the vagina to the lower abdominal wall, to the ligaments of the pelvis (sacrospinous ligaments), or to the lower back spine.

How invasive is this surgery?

The sacral colpopexy procedure is moderately invasive and is done under general anesthesia. This surgery can be approached using vaginal or abdominal (open or laparoscopic) incisions. As with other prolapse procedures, sacral colpopexy is often performed with other prolapse repairs, urinary incontinence surgeries, or hysterectomies. Most patients recover after a day or two in the hospital and might go home with a catheter. The length of the surgery in addition to the general anesthesia and recovery time make this procedure moderately invasive.

How is this surgery performed?

During a vaginal vault repair, an incision is made in the anterior (front) abdominal wall. Then a tunnel is usually created through the peritoneum (the large membrane in the abdominal cavity that supports the internal organs) to the vaginal vault and sacral promontory (a jutting portion on the roof of the pelvic cavity). The vaginal apex is then raised and repositioned, usually by attaching it to the sacrospinous pelvic ligaments.

This procedure can also be performed transvaginally or laparoscopically, via several small abdominal incisions. Some surgeons have special training in using a robotic device called the Da Vinci robot (manufactured by Intuitive Surgical) to perform sacral colpopexy. With this device, the surgeon is seated at a console a few feet away from the patient and operates miniaturized surgical instruments using the console. The console sends augmented three-dimensional images of the surgical field back to the surgeon. The Da Vinci robot is FDA approved for this procedure and is minimally invasive. The Da Vinci robot has even been used in operations when the surgeon is located on a separate continent from the patient, although this is not the main purpose or focus of the device.

What are the success rates of this surgery?

The sacral colpopexy procedure appears to be effective in providing durable support of the vaginal vault in up to 97 percent of women who have the surgery.[42] Women had better success rates with the abdominal approach than the transvaginal approach, with 85 percent of women satisfied with the abdominal approach and 81 percent satisfied with the transvaginal approach. The abdominal approach is less likely to result in postsurgical anterior vaginal wall prolapse and postoperative vault prolapse.[43]

Uterine Suspension Procedures

Uterine suspension procedures correct uterine prolapse (when the uterus falls or slides from its normal position into the vagina). Uterine prolapse happens when the muscles, ligaments, and other supporting pelvic structures that hold the uterus in place weaken. This kind of prolapse often occurs with cystoceles, rectoceles, and enteroceles.

Uterine suspension surgeries reposition the uterus by lifting it and attaching it to nearby ligaments. Because these suspension procedures do not remove the uterus (as a hysterectomy does), they are a good choice for women who wish to have children in the future. The preservation of a woman's uterus can also have positive psychological benefits.[44] The suspension procedures can be performed abdominally, vaginally, or laparoscopically. Success rates for uterine suspension vary, ranging from 73 percent to 100 percent, depending on the chosen approach.[45] These procedures are often performed at the same time as other pelvic organ prolapse repairs.

Hysterectomy

Hysterectomy is a much more radical approach to correcting uterine prolapse, removing a portion of or the entire uterus. Depending on the severity of the uterine prolapse, as well as the presence of other health conditions or additional pelvic organ prolapses, the surgeon may choose to remove only the upper part of the uterus; the entire uterus and cervix; or the entire uterus, cervix, and top of the vagina. The last option is usually reserved for the treatment of cancer.

A hysterectomy can be performed abdominally, as an open procedure, or less invasively through the vagina or via laparoscopy.[46] Since this surgical procedure completely removes the prolapsed uterus, the cure rate is 100 percent.[47] This surgery is often performed in conjunction with other pelvic organ repair procedures.

Sacral Neuromodulation

What is sacral neuromodulation?

In the sacral neuromodulation procedure, the surgeon implants a small device under the skin that uses a mild electrical current to stimulate the sacral nerve. The goal of this sacral nerve stimulation is to address the urge and frequency associated with overactive bladder, urge incontinence, and urge-dominant mixed urinary incontinence. This device also helps women who experience urinary leakage from urge incontinence as well as women who have nonobstructive urinary retention (which means they have difficulty urinating but no blockage in the bladder or urethra).

Who are ideal candidates for this surgery?

Sacral neuromodulation is ideal for women whose symptoms have not responded to conservative therapies. This surgery is not appropriate for women who do not have the mental or physical ability to operate the settings on the neurostimulator, which controls the implanted device. This procedure is also not recommended for women who do not respond well to the stimulator in a presurgical test situation.

How does this surgery work?

Because the conditions addressed by sacral neuromodulation are usually caused by faulty communication between the nerves, brain, and bladder, the implanted device works by restoring order to those communication pathways. Research shows that stimulating the sacral nerve reduces involuntary contractions of the bladder and helps to regulate the voiding reflex.[48] The device can be set so that bladder contractions occur on a preset schedule.

How invasive is this surgery?

Sacral neuromodulation is minimally invasive and usually performed as an outpatient procedure. The surgery can be performed under general anesthesia or under local anesthesia with sedation.

How is this surgery performed?

During the procedure, the surgeon implants a device that sends mild electrical pulses to nerves that control the bladder, pelvic organs, and pelvic floor muscles. The tiny device is flat and usually measures less than two and a half inches. It is usually implanted under the skin in the buttock. A thin lead wire is then anchored near the sacral nerve so that the electrical pulses can stimulate the relevant pelvic nerves.

What are the success rates for this surgery?

For women who have the urgency and frequency associated with overactive bladder, sacral neuromodulation provides a cure for 31 percent. A further 33 percent of women who underwent the procedure reported an improvement in symptoms. For women with urinary leakage from urge incontinence, this surgery provides a cure for up to 65 percent,[49] and a further 34 percent experience an improvement in symptoms.[50] Sacral neuromodulation has a success rate of 33 to 79 percent for women suffering from chronic nonobstructive urinary retention.[51]

Additional Resources

The more knowledge you have about your condition, the better you can advocate for your health. Consult our website for updates, ongoing developments, and more. Plus, read our blog and follow us on Twitter. Find us online at these sites:

Website: www.awomansguidetopelvichealth.com
Twitter: twitter.com/#!/wetmatters

Learn more about the different types of incontinence, pelvic organ prolapses, as well as decreased sexual sensation by using the additional resources listed below.

American Academy of Family Physicians
P.O. Box 11210
Shawnee Mission, KS 66207-1210
800-274-2237 or 913-906-6000
www.aafp.org/afp/20000701/127.html

American Association of Sexuality Educators, Counselors and Therapists
P.O. Box 1960
Ashland, VA 23005
804-752-0026
www.aasect.org

American College of Obstetricians and Gynecologists
P.O. Box 96920
409 12th Street SW
Washington, DC 20090-6920
202-863-2518
www.acog.org (search for "Urinary incontinence")

American Physical Therapy Association
Section on Women's Health
P.O. Box 327
Alexandria, VA 22313
800-999-APTA, ext. 3229
www.womenshealthapta.org

American Urological Association Foundation
1000 Corporate Boulevard
Linthicum, MD 21090
1-866-746-4282 (toll free, U.S. only)
www.urologyhealth.org

MedlinePlus
National Library of Medicine
8600 Rockville Pike
Bethesda, MD 20894
1-888-FIND-NLM or 301-594-5983
www.nlm.nih.gov/medlineplus/femalesexualdysfunction.html
www.nlm.nih.gov/medlineplus/urinaryincontinence.html

National Association for Continence
P.O. Box 1019
Charleston, SC 29402-1019
1-800-BLADDER or 843-377-0900
www.nafc.org/media/media-kit/facts-statistics

National Institutes of Health State-of-the-Science Conference Statement:
Prevention of Fecal and Urinary Incontinence in Adults, *Annals of Internal Medicine*
www.annals.org/cgi/content/full/148/6/449

National Kidney and Urologic Diseases Clearinghouse
3 Information Way
Bethesda, MD 20892-3580
1-800-891-5390
www.kidney.niddk.nih.gov/Kudiseases/pubs/uiwomen/index.htm

North American Menopause Society
5900 Landerbrook Drive, Suite 390
Mayfield Heights, OH 44124
440-442-7550
www.menopause.org

Sexuality Information and Education Council of the United States
90 John Street, Suite 704
New York, NY 10038
212-819-9770
www.siecus.org

Society for Sex Therapy and Research
409 12th Street SW
Washington, DC 20090-6920
202-863-1648
www.sstarnet.org

Society for the Scientific Study of Sexuality
P.O. Box 416
Allentown, PA 18105-0416
610-443-3100
www.sexscience.org

UroToday
1802 Fifth Street
Berkeley, CA 94710
510-540-0930 (fax)
info@urotoday.com
www.urotoday.com/stress-urinary-incontinence-1483.html

References

Chapter 1. Anatomy and Pelvic Floor Health

1. Rackley, R., Firoozi, F. 2009. Injectable Bulking Agents for Incontinence. *Medscape.* http://emedicine.medscape.com/article/447068-overview (accessed 5/26/11).

Chapter 2. Stress Urinary Incontinence

1. Brigham and Women's Hospital. 2011. Urinary Incontinence. *U.S. News and World Report.* http://health.usnews.com/health-conditions/urology/urinary-incontinence/overview (accessed 5/26/11).

2. Muller, N. 2005. What Americans understand and how they are affected by bladder control problems: Highlights of recent nationwide consumer research. *Urologic Nursing* 25 (2): 109-15.

3. Subak, L. L., Brubaker, L., Chai, T. C., Creasman, J. M., Diokno, A. C., Goode, P. S., Kraus, S. R., Kusek, J. W., Leng, W. W., Lukacz, E. S., Norton, P., Tennstedt, S., Urinary Incontinence Treatment Network. 2008. High costs of urinary incontinence among women electing surgery to treat stress incontinence. *Obstet Gynecol.* 1111 (4): 899-907.

4. Rapp, D. E., Kobashi, K. C. 2008. Mid-urethral slings: Techniques and outcomes. *Urology Times—Clinical Edition* (Aug. 1).

5. Brigham and Women's Hospital. 2011. Urinary Incontinence.

6. Subak, L. L., Wing, R., West, D. S., Franklin, F., Vittinghoff, E., Creasman, J. M., Richter, H. E., Myers, D., Burgio, K. L., Gorin, A. A., Macer, J., Kusek, J. W., Grady, D., PRIDE Investigators. 2009. Weight loss to treat urinary incontinence in overweight and obese women. *N Engl J Med.* 360 (5): 481-90.

7. Muller, N. 2005. What Americans understand.

8. Cullen, P. J., Heit, M. 2000. Urinary incontinence in women: Evaluation and management. *Am Fam Phys.* 1;62 (11): 2433-44.

9. Subak, L. L., Van Den Eeden, S., Thom, D., Creasman, J. M., Brown, J. S., Re-

productive Risks for Incontinence Study at Kaiser (RRISK) Research Group. 2007. Urinary incontinence in women: Direct costs of routine care. *Am J Obstet Gynecol.* 197: 1-9.

10. Agency for Health Care Policy and Research. 1996. Overview: Urinary Incontinence in Adults, Clinical Practice Guideline Update. www.ahrq.gov/clinic/uiovervw.htm (accessed 5/26/11).

11. Denson, M., Houser, E. 2006. *Improving the Symptoms and Quality of Life of Patients with Overactive Bladder and Urinary Incontinence.* Brochure. The Urology Team, PA.

12. Bo, K., Talseth, T., Holme, I. 1999. Single blind, randomised controlled trial of pelvic floor exercises, electrical stimulation, vaginal cones, and no treatment in management of genuine stress incontinence in women. *BMJ* 318: 487-93.

13. Neumann, P. B., Grimmer, K. A., Deenadayalan, Y. 2006. Pelvic floor muscle training and adjunctive therapies for the treatment of stress urinary incontinence in women: A systematic review. *BMC Women's Health.* www.medscape.com/viewarticle/548855 (accessed 5/26/11).

14. Paddison, K. 2002. Complying with pelvic floor exercises: A literature review. *Nursing Standard* 16 (39): 33–38.

15. Freidman, R. 2002. Electrical stimulation effective for urinary incontinence. Presented at the American Urogynecologic Society. Doctor's Guide. www.docguide.com/news/content.nsf/news/8525697700573E1885256C590071D6C0 (accessed 5/26/11).

16. Davila, G. W., Ghoniem, G. M., Wexner, S. D., eds. 2010. *Pelvic Floor Dysfunction: A Multidisciplinary Approach.* London: Springer.

17. Gillenwater, J. Y. 1991. *Adult and Pediatric Urology.* St. Louis: Mosby Year Book.

18. Daniels, R. 2008. *Nursing Fundamentals: Caring and Clinical Decision Making.* Clifton Park, NY: Delmar Cengage Learning.

19. Mayo Clinic Staff. 2009. Bladder Control Problems: Medications for Treating Urinary Incontinence. www.mayoclinic.com/health/bladder-control-problems/w000123 (accessed 5/26/11).

20. National Institutes of Health, Medline Plus. 2009. Stress Incontinence. www.nlm.nih.gov/medlineplus/ency/article/000891.htm (accessed 5/26/11).

21. National Association for Continence. 2010. Non-surgical Treatments for Female Stress Urinary Incontinence. www.nafc.org/bladder-bowel-health/types-of-incontinence/stress-incontinence/non-surgical-treatment-for-female-stress-urinary-incontinence/#6 (accessed 5/26/11).

22. Subak et al. 2009. Weight loss.

23. Schmidt, J. 2007. Acupuncture and Tai Chi as Incontinence Treatments. In continenceNetwork.com. www.healthcentral.com/incontinence/c/45/10980/tai-chi/ (accessed 5/26/11).

24. Kocjancic, E., Crivellaro, S., Oyama, I. A., Singla, A., Ranzoni, S., Carone, R., Manassero, A., Gontero, P., Frea, B. 2008. Transobturator tape in the management

of female stress incontinence: Clinical outcomes at medium-term follow-up. *Urol Int.* 80 (3): 275-78.

25. Mitsui, T., Tanaka, H., Moriya, K., Kakizaki, H., Nonomura, K. 2007. Clinical and urodynamic outcomes of pubovaginal sling procedure with autologous rectus fascia for stress urinary incontinence. *Int J of Urol.* 14 (2): 1076-79.

Chapter 3. Overactive Bladder and Urge Urinary Incontinence

1. Stewart, W. F., Van Rooyen, J. B., Cundiff, G. W., Abrams, P., Herzog, A. R., Corey, R., Hunt, T. L., Wein, A. J. 2003. Prevalence and burden of overactive bladder in the United States. *World J Urol.* 20: 327-36.

2. Stoddard, H., Donovan, J., Whitley, E., Sharp, D., Harvey, I. 2001. Urinary incontinence in older people in the community: A neglected problem? *Br J Ger Pract.* 51: 548-52. Hannestad, Y. S., Rortveit, G., Hunskaar, S. 2002. Help-seeking and associated factors in female urinary incontinence: The Norwegian EPINCONT study. *Scand J Prim Health Care* 20: 102-107.

3. Cullen, P. J., Heit, M. 2000. Urinary incontinence in women: Evaluation and management. *Am Fam Phys.* 1;62 (11): 2433-44.

4. Abrams, P., Cardozo, L., Fall, M., Griffiths, D., Rosier, P., Ulmsten, U., van Kerrebroeck, P., Victor, A., Wein, A., Standardisation Sub-committee of the International Continence Society. 2002. The standardisation of terminology of lower urinary tract function: Report from the Standardisation Sub-committee for the International Continence Society. *Neurourol Urodyn.* 21: 167-78.

5. Stewart et al. 2003. Prevalence and burden.

6. Ibid. Elving, L. B., Foldspang, A., Lam, G. W., Mommsen, S. 1989. Descriptive epidemiology of urinary incontinence in 3,100 women aged 30-59. *Scan J Urol Nephrol Suppl.* 125: 37-43. Bo, K., Borgen, J. S. 2001. Prevalence of stress and urge urinary incontinence in elite athletes and controls. *Med Sci Sports Exerc.* 33 (11): 1797-1802.

7. National Institute of Diabetes and Digestive and Kidney Diseases. 2007. Urinary incontinence in women. *NIH Publications* 8 (4132): 3.

8. Stewart et al. 2003. Prevalence and burden.

9. Cullen and Heit. 2000. Urinary incontinence.

10. Milsom, I., Stewart, W., Thüroff, J. 1999. The prevalence of overactive bladder. Presented at the 14th Congress of the European Association of Gynecology and Obstetrics. (Sept.) Granada, Spain.

11. Ricci, J. A., Baggish, J. S., Hunt, T. L., Stewart, W. F., Wein, A., Herzog, A. R., Diokno, A. 2001. Coping strategies and health care-seeking behavior in a U.S. national sample of adults with symptoms suggestive of overactive bladder. *Clin Ther.* 23: 1245-59. Shaw, C., Tansey, R., Jackson, C., Hyde, C., Allan, R. 2001. Barriers to help seeking in people with urinary symptoms. *Fam Pract.* 18: 48-52.

12. Stach-Lempinen, B., Hakala, A. L., Laippala, P., Lehtinen, K., Metsänoja, R.,

Kujansuu, E. 2003. Severe depression determines quality of life in urinary incontinent women. *Neurourol Urodyn.* 22: 563-68. Darkow, T., Fontes, C. L., Williamson, T. E. 2005. Costs associated with the management of overactive bladder and related comorbidities. *Pharmacotherapy* 25: 511-19.

13. Hu, T-W., Wagner, T. H., Bentkover, J. D., LeBlanc, K., Zhou, S. Z., Hunt, T. 2004. Cost of urinary incontinence and overactive bladder in the United States: A comparative study. *Urology* 63: 461-65.

14. Agency for Health Care Policy and Research. 1996. Overview: Urinary Incontinence in Adults, Clinical Practice Guideline Update. www.ahrq.gov/clinic/uiover vw.htm (accessed 5/26/11).

15. National Institutes of Health, Medline Plus. 2011. Urge Incontinence. www.nm .nih.gov/medlineplus/ency/article/001270.htm (accessed 5/26/11).

16. Hay-Smith, E. J., Berghmans, L. C. M., Hendriks, H. J. M. 2003. Pelvic floor muscle training for urinary incontinence in women [Cochrane review]. In *Cochrane Library* 1. Chichester: John Wiley and Sons. Wyman, J. F., Fantl, J. A., McClish, D. K., Bump, R. C. 1998. Comparative efficacy of behavioral interventions in the management of female urinary incontinence. *Am J Obstet Gynecol.* 179: 999-1007.

17. Yamanishi, T., Yasuda, K., Sakakibara, R., Hattori, T., Suda, S. 2000. Randomized double-blind study of electrical stimulation for urinary incontinence due to detrusor activity. *Urology* 55: 353-57.

18. Freidman, R. 2002. Electrical stimulation effective for urinary incontinence. Presented at the American Urogynecologic Society. Doctor's Guide. www.docguide.com/ news/content.nsf/news/8525697700573E1885256C590071D6C0 (accessed 5/26/11).

19. Diokno, A. C., Appell, R. A., Sand, P. K., Dmochowski, R. R., Gburek, B. M., Klimberg, I. W., Kell, S. H., OPERA Study Group. 2003. Prospective, randomized, double-blind study of the efficacy and tolerability of the extended-release formulations of oxybutynin and tolterodine for overactive bladder: Results of the OPERA trial. *Mayo Clin Proc.* 78: 687-95.

20. Moehrer, B., Hextall, A., Jackson, S. 2003. Oestrogens for urinary incontinence in women [review]. *Cochrane Database Syst Rev.* 2.

21. Subak, L. L., Wing, R., West, D. S., Franklin, F., Vittinghoff, E., Creasman, J. M., Richter, H. E., Myers, D., Burgio, K. L., Gorin, A. A., Macer, J., Kusek, J. W., Grady, D., PRIDE Investigators. 2009. Weight loss to treat urinary incontinence in overweight and obese women. *N Engl J Med.* 360 (5): 481-90.

22. Graham, P., Cook, T. 2008. Acupuncture for the treatment of overactive bladder. *Journal of the Association of Chartered Physiotherapists in Women's Health* 102: 53-58.

23. Bergström, K., Carlsson, C. P., Lindholm, C., Widengren, R. 2000. Improvement of urge- and mixed-type incontinence after acupuncture treatment among elderly women—a pilot study. *Journal of the Autonomic Nervous System* 79 (2-3): 173-80.

24. Amundsen, C. L., Romero, A. A., Jamison, M. G., Webster, G. D. 2008. Sacral neuromodulation for intractable urge incontinence: Are there factors associated

with cure? *Urology* 66 (4): 363. Van Kerrebroeck, P., van Voskuilen, A. C., Heesakkers, J. P., Lycklama à Nijeholt, A. A., Siegel, S., Jonas, U., Fowler, C. J., Fall, M., Gajewski, J. B., Hassouna, M. M., Cappellano, F., Elhilali, M. M., Milam, D. F., Das, A. K., Dijkema, H. E., van den Hombergh, U. 2007. Results of sacral neuromodulation therapy for urinary voiding dysfunctions: Outcomes of a prospective, worldwide clinical study. *J Urol.* 178: 2029-34.

Chapter 4. Mixed Urinary Incontinence

1. Sandvik, H., Hunskaar, S., Vanvik, A., Bratt, H., Seim, A., Hermstad, R. 1995. Diagnostic classification of female urinary incontinence: An epidemiological survey corrected for validity. *J Clin Epidemiol.* 48: 339-43. Hannestad, Y. S., Rortveit, G., Sandvik, H., Hunskaar, S., Norwegian EPINCONT study. Epidemiology of Incontinence in the County of Nord-Trøndelag. 2000. A community-based epidemiological survey of female urinary incontinence: The Norwegian EPINCONT study. *J Clin Epidemiol.* 53: 1150-57.

2. Bump, R. C., Norton, P. A., Zinner, N. R., Yalcin, I., Duloxetine Urinary Incontinence Study Group. 2003. Mixed urinary incontinence symptoms: Urodynamic findings, incontinence severity, and treatment response. *Obstet Gynecol.* 102: 76-83.

3. Smith, P. P., McCrery, R. J., Appell, R. A. 2006. Current trends in the evaluation and management of female urinary incontinence. *CMAJ* 175 (10): 1233-40.

4. Hannestad et al. 2000. Norwegian EPINCONT study.

5. Sandvik et al. 1995. Diagnostic classification of female urinary incontinence. Weidner, A. C., Myers, E. R., Visco, A. G., Cundiff, G. W., Bump, R. C. 2001. Which women with stress incontinence require urodynamics? *Am J Obstet Gynecol.* 184: 20-27.

6. Bump et al. 2003. Mixed urinary incontinence symptoms.

7. Javachandran, C. 2007. Prevalence of stress, urge, and mixed urinary incontinence in women. *Masters Theses and Doctoral Dissertations.* Paper 228. Eastern Michigan University.

8. Abrams, P., Cardozo, L., Fall, M., Griffiths, D., Rosier, P., Ulmsten, U., van Kerrebroeck, P., Victor, A., Wein, A., Standardisation Sub-committee of the International Continence Society. 2002. The standardisation of terminology of lower urinary tract function: Report from the Standardisation Sub-committee for the International Continence Society. *Neurourol Urodyn.* 21: 167-78.

9. Bump et al. 2003. Mixed urinary incontinence symptoms.

10. Ibid.

11. Subak L. L., Van Den Eeden, S., Thom, D., Creasman, J. M., Brown, J. S., Reproductive Risks for Incontinence Study at Kaiser (RRISK) Research Group. 2007. Urinary incontinence in women: Direct costs of routine care. *Am J Obstet Gynecol.* 197: 1-9.

12. Mahajan, S. T., Elkadry, E. A., Kenton, K. S., Shott, S., Brubaker, L. 2006. Patient-centered surgical outcomes: The impact of goal achievement and urge in-

continence on patient satisfaction one year after surgery. *Am J Obstet Gynecol.* 194 (3): 722-28.

Chapter 5. Pelvic Organ Prolapse

1. Nygaard, I., Bradley, C., Brandt, D., Women's Health Initiative. 2004. Pelvic organ prolapse in older women: Prevalence and risk factors. *Obstet Gynecol.* 104: 489-97. Rortveit, G., Brown, J. S., Thom, D. H., Van Den Eeden, S. K., Creasman, J. M., Subak, L. L. 2007. Symptomatic pelvic organ prolapse: Prevalence and risk factors in a population-based, racially diverse cohort. *Obstet Gynecol.* 109: 1396-1403.

2. Samuelson, E. C., Victor, F. T., Tibblin, G., Svärdsudd, K. F. 1999. Signs of genital prolapse in a Swedish population of women 20 to 59 years of age and possible related factors. *Am J Obstet Gynecol.* 180: 299-305. Swift, S., Woodman, P., O'Boyle, A., Kahn, M., Valley, M., Bland, D., Wang, W., Schaffer, J. 2005. Pelvic Organ Support Study (POSST): The distribution, clinical definition, and epidemiologic condition of pelvic organ support defects. *Am J Gynecol.* 192: 795-806.

3. Mayo Clinic Staff. 2010 (a). Kegel Exercises: A How-to Guide for Women. *Mayo Foundation for Medical Education and Research.* www.mayoclinic.com/health/kegel -exercises/WO00119 (accessed 5/26/11).

4. Mayo Clinic Staff. 2010 (b). Uterine Prolapse: Preparing for Your Appointment. *Mayo Foundation for Medical Education and Research.* www.mayoclinic.com/health/ uterine-prolapse/DS00700/DSECTION=preparing-for-your-appointment (accessed 5/26/11).

5. Saint Louis University. 2008. Family history places women at risk of pelvic organ prolapse. *ScienceDaily.* www.sciencedaily.com/releases/2008/04/080430172800.htm (accessed 5/26/11).

6. Olsen, A. L., Smith, V. J., Bergstrom, J. O., Colling, J. C., Clark, A. L. 1997. Epidemiology of surgically managed pelvic organ prolapse and urinary incontinence. *Obstet Gynecol.* 89: 501-506.

7. Samuelson et al. 1999. Signs of genital prolapse.

8. Kuncharapu, I., Majeroni, B., Johnson, D. 2010. Pelvic organ prolapse. *Am Fam Phys.* 81: 9. Hendrix, S. L., Clark, A., Nygaard, I., Aragaki, A., Barnabei, V., McTiernan, A. 2002. Pelvic organ prolapse in the Women's Health Initiative: Gravity and gravidy. *Am J Gynecol.* 186: 1160-66.

9. Kuncharapu et al. 2010. Pelvic organ prolapse.

10. Mant, J., Painter, R., Vessey, M. 1997. Epidemiology of genital prolapse: Observations from the Oxford Family Planning Association Study. *Br J Obstet Gynaecol.* 104: 579-85.

11. Handa, V. L. 2003. Report from the 24th Annual Scientific Meeting of the American Urogynecological Society. *Medscape Ob/Gyn & Women's Health* 8: 2. www.med scape.com/viewarticle/461719_print (accessed 5/26/11).

12. Burrows, L. J., Shaw, H. 2008. Contemporary management of pelvic organ prolapse. *Menopause Management* (Sept.-Oct.): 23-30.

13. Strohbehn, K., Jakary, J. A., DeLancey, J. O. 1997. Pelvic organ prolapse in young women. *Obstet Gynecol.* 90: 33-36.

14. Tinelli, A., Malvasi, A., Rahimi, S., Negro, R., Vergara, D., Martignago, R., Pellegrino, M., Cavallotti, C. 2010. Age-related pelvic floor modifications and prolapse risk factors in postmenopausal women. *Menopause* 17 (1): 204-12.

15. Eunice Kennedy Shriver National Institute of Child Health and Human Development. 2010. Pelvic Floor Disorders. *National Institutes of Health.* www.nichd.nih .gov/health/topics/pelvic_floor_disorders.cfm.

16. Mayo Clinic Staff 2010 (a). Kegel Exercises.

17. Denson, M., Houser, E. 2006. *Treatment Plan for Pelvic Floor Prolapse.* Brochure. The Urology Team, PA.

18. Mayo Clinic Staff 2010 (b). Uterine Prolapse.

19. Hagen, S., Stark, D., Maher, C., Adams, E. 2006. Conservative management of pelvic organ prolapse in women. *Cochrane Database Sys. Rev.* 2.

20. Mayo Clinic Staff 2010 (a). Kegel Exercises.

21. Burrows and Shaw. 2008. Contemporary management.

22. Bump, R. C., Norton, P. A. 1998. Epidemiology and natural history of pelvic floor dysfunction. *Obstet Gynecol Clinics North America* 4: 723-46.

23. Brincat, C., Kenton, K., FitzGerald, M. P., Brubaker, L. 2004. Sexual activity predicts continued pessary use. *Am J Obstet Gynecol.* 191: 198-200.

24. Burrows and Shaw. 2008. Contemporary management.

25. Cundiff, G. W., Amundsen, C. L., Bent, A. E., Coates, K. W., Schaffer, J. I., Strohbehn, K., Handa, V. L. 2007. The PESSRI study: Symptom relief outcomes of a randomized crossover trial of the ring and Gellhorn pessaries. *Am J Obstet Gynecol.* 197: 405.

26. Fernando, R. J., Thakar, R., Sultan, A. H., Shah, S. M., Jones, P. W. 2006. Effect of vaginal pessaries on symptoms associated with pelvic organ prolapse. *Obstet Gynecol.* 108: 93.

27. Sulak, P. J., Kuehl, T. J., Shull, B. L. 1993. Vaginal pessaries and their use in pelvic relaxation. *J Reprod Med.* 38: 919-23.

28. Clark, A. L., Gregory, T., Smith, V. J., Edwards, R. 2003. Epidemiological evaluation of reoperation for surgically treated pelvic organ prolapse and urinary incontinence. *Am J Obstet Gynecol.* 189: 1261-67.

Chapter 6. Decreased Sexual Sensation

1. Meston, C. M., Hull, E., Levin, R. J., Sipski, M. 2004. Disorders of orgasm in women. *J Sex Med.* 1 (1): 66-68.

2. Weston, L. C. 2008. Can't orgasm? Here's help for women. *WebMD the Magazine* (March-April). www.webmd.com/sex-relationships/features/cant-orgasm-heres -help-for-women (accessed 5/26/11).

3. National Institutes of Health, Medline Plus. 2010. Orgasmic Dysfunction. www .nlm.nih.gov/medlineplus/ency/article/001953.htm (accessed 5/26/11).

4. Davison, S. L., Bell, R. J., La China, M., Holden, S. L., Davis, S. R. 2008. Sexual function in well women: Stratification by sexual satisfaction, hormone use, and menopause status. *J Sex Med.* 5 (5): 1214-22.

5. Arias, E., MacDorman, M. F., Strobino, D. M., Guyer, B. 2003. Annual summary of vital statistics—2002. *Pediatrics* 112: 1215-30.

6. Waterstone, M., Wolfe, C., Hooper, R., Bewley, S. 2003. Postnatal morbidity after childbirth and severe obstetric morbidity. *BJOG* 110: 128-33.

7. Ibid.

8. Ibid.

9. Ibid.

10. Gorman, M. O. 2009. Good Sex Gives Women a Sense of a Higher Purpose. *Rodale News: Prevention Healthy Living Group.* www.rodale.com/sexual-satisfaction -women?page=0%2C0 (accessed 5/26/11).

11. Davison, S. L., Bell, R. J., La China, M., Holden, S. L., Davis, S. R. 2009. The relationship between self-reported sexual satisfaction and general well-being in women. *J Sex Med.* 6 (10): 2690-97.

12. Bradford, A., Meston, C. M. 2010. Behavior and symptom change among women treated with placebo for sexual dysfunction. *J Sex Med.* 8 (1): 191-201.

13. Connell, K., Guess, M. K., La Combe, J., Wang, A., Powers, K., Lazarou, G., Mikhail, M. 2005. Evaluation of the role of pudendal nerve integrity in female sexual function using noninvasive techniques. *Am J Obstet Gynecol.* 192 (5): 1712-17.

14. Davison et al. 2008. Sexual function in well women.

15. Center for Sexual Health Promotion, Indiana University. 2010. Results of the National Survey of Sexual Health and Behavior (NSSHB). *J Sex Med.* 7 (5): 243-373.

16. Getliffe, K., and Dolman, M. 2007. *Promoting Continence: A Clinical and Research Resource.* Oxford, UK: Bailliere Tindall.

17. Ibid.

18. Torpy, J. M. 2007. Women's sexual concerns after menopause. *JAMA* 297 (6): 664.

19. Guess, M., Connell, K., Schrader, S., Reutman, S., Wang, A., LaCombe, J., Toennis, C., Lowe, B., Melman, A., Mikhail, M. 2006. Decreased genital sensation in competitive women cyclists. *J Sex Med.* 3 (6): 949-1101.

20. Jozwik, M. 1998. The physiological basis of pelvic floor exercises in the treatment of stress urinary incontinence. *BJOG* 105: 1046-51.

21. Women's Sexual Health Foundation. August 20, 2007. Women's Sexual Health Survey: 91% of healthcare providers are not regularly asking patients about sexual health difficulties. Press release. Cincinnati, OH: Women's Sexual Health Foundation.

22. Klein, M. C., Gauthier, R. J., Robbins, J. M., Kaczorowski, J., Jorgensen, S. H., Franco, E. D., Johnson, B., Waghorn, K., Gelfand, M. M., Guralnick, M. S., et al. 1994. Relationship of episiotomy to perineal trauma and morbidity, sexual dysfunction, and pelvic floor relaxation. *Am J Obstet Gynecol.* 171: 591-98. Glazener, C. M. 1997.

Sexual function after childbirth: Women's experiences, persistent morbidity, and lack of professional morbidity. *BJOG* 104: 330-35.

23. Beji, N. K., Yalcin, O., Erkan, H. A. 2003. The effect of pelvic floor training on sexual function of treated patients. *Int Urogynecol J Pelvic Floor Dysfunct.* 14: 234-38.

24. Muller, N. 2005. Keeping the vital pelvic floor healthy. *J Active Aging* (May-June): 34-36.

25. Rivalta, M., Sighinolfi, M. C., De Stefani, S., Micali, S., Mofferdin, A., Grande, M., Bianchi, G. 2009. Biofeedback, electrical stimulation, pelvic floor muscle exercises, and vaginal cones: A combined rehabilitative approach for sexual dysfunction associated with urinary incontinence. *J Sex Med.* 6 (6): 1674-77.

26. Dean, N., Wilson, D., Herbison, P., Glazener, C., Aung, T., Macarthur, C. 2008. Sexual function, delivery mode history, pelvic floor muscle exercises and incontinence: A cross-sectional study six years post-partum. *Aust NZ J Obstet Gynaecol.* 48 (3): 302-11.

27. Bump, R. C., Norton, P. A. 1998. Epidemiology and natural history of pelvic floor dysfunction. *Obstet Gynecol Clinics North America* 4: 723-46.

28. Subak, L. L., Wing, R., West, D. S., Franklin, F., Vittinghoff, E., Creasman, J. M., Richter, H. E., Myers, D., Burgio, K. L., Gorin, A. A., Macer, J., Kusek, J. W., Grady, D., PRIDE Investigators. 2009. Weight loss to treat urinary incontinence in overweight and obese women. *N Engl J Med.* 360 (5): 481-90.

29. Mayo Clinic Staff. 2009. Bladder Control Problems: Medications for Treating Urinary Incontinence. www.mayoclinic.com/health/bladder-control-problems/w000123 (accessed 5/26/11).

Chapter 7. At-Home Pelvic Floor Muscle Exercise Program

1. Bo, K., Talseth, T., Holme, I. 1999. Single blind, randomised controlled trial of pelvic floor exercises, electrical stimulation, vaginal cones, and no treatment in management of genuine stress incontinence in women. *BMJ* 318:487-93.

2. Bump, R. C., Norton, P. A. 1998. Epidemiology and natural history of pelvic floor dysfunction. *Obstet Gynecol Clinics North America* 4: 723-46.

3. Bo, K. 2003. Is there still a place for physiotherapy in the treatment of female incontinence? *EAU Update Series* 1: 145-53.

4. Kincade, J. E., Dougherty, M. C., Busby-Whitehead, J., Carlson, J. R., Nix, W. B., Kelsey, D. T., Smith, F. C., Hunter, G. S., Rix, A. D. 2005. Self-monitoring and pelvic floor muscle exercises to treat urinary incontinence. *Urol Nurs.* 25 (5): 353-63.

5. Kincade et al. 2005. Self-monitoring. Bo, K., Kvarstein, B., Nygaard, I. 2005. Lower urinary tract symptoms and pelvic floor muscle exercise adherence after 15 years. *Obstet Gynecol.* 105 (5): 999-1005.

6. Bump, R. C., Hurt, W. G., Fantl, J. A., Wyman, J. F. 1991. Assessment of Kegel pelvic muscle exercise performance after brief verbal instruction. *Am J Obstet Gynecol.* 165: 322-29.

7. Bo, K. 2004. Pelvic floor muscle training is effective in treatment of female

stress urinary incontinence, but how does it work? *Int Urogynecol J Pelvic Floor Dysfunct.* 15: 76–84.

8. Bo et al. 1999. Single blind, randomised controlled trial. Morkved, S., Bo, K., Fjortoft, T. 2002. Effect of adding biofeedback to pelvic floor muscle training to treat urodynamic stress incontinence. *Obstet Gynecol.* 100: 730–39.

9. Neumann, P. B., Grimmer, K. A., Deenadayalan, Y. 2006. Pelvic floor muscle training and adjunctive therapies for the treatment of stress urinary incontinence in women: A systematic review. *BMC Women's Health.* www.medscape.com/view article/548855 (accessed 5/26/11).

10. Nygaard, I. E. 1996. Nonoperative management of urinary incontinence. *Current Opinion in Obstetrics and Gynecology* 8: 15. Burgio, K. L., Locher, J. L., Goode, P. S., Hardin, J. M., McDowell, B. J., Dombrowski, M., Candib, D. 1998. Behavioral vs. drug treatment for urge urinary incontinence in older women in a randomized controlled trial. *JAMA* 280: 1995–2000.

11. Hagen, S., Stark, D., Maher, C., Adams, E. 2006. Conservative management of pelvic organ prolapse in women. *Cochrane Database Sys.* Oct 18 (4): CD003882. Mayo Clinic Staff. 2010. Kegel Exercises: A How-to Guide for Women. *Mayo Foundation for Medical Education and Research.* www.mayoclinic.com/health/kegel-exercises/ WO00119 (accessed 5/26/11).

12. Braekken, I. H., Majida, M., Engh, M. E., Bo, K. 2010. Morphological changes after pelvic floor muscle training measured by 3-dimensional ultrasonography: A randomized controlled trial. *Obstet Gynecol.* 115 (2, pt. 1): 317–24.

13. Dean, N., Wilson, D., Herbison, P., Glazener, C., Aung, T., Macarthur, C. 2008. Sexual function, delivery mode history, pelvic floor muscle exercises and incontinence: A cross-sectional study six years post-partum. *Aust NZ J Obstet Gynaecol.* 48 (3): 302–11.

14. Glazener, C. M. 1997. Sexual function after childbirth: Women's experiences, persistent morbidity, and lack of professional morbidity. *BJOG* 104: 330–35.

15. Rivalta, M., Sighinolfi, M. C., De Stefani, S., Micali, S., Mofferdin, A., Grande, M., Bianchi, G. 2009. Biofeedback, electrical stimulation, pelvic floor muscle exercises, and vaginal cones: A combined rehabilitative approach for sexual dysfunction associated with urinary incontinence. *J Sex Med.* 6 (6): 1674–77.

16. Beji, N. K., Yalcin, O., Erkan, H. A. 2003. The effect of pelvic floor training on sexual function of treated patients. *Int Urogynecol J Pelvic Floor Dysfunct.* 14: 234–38.

17. American College of Sports Medicine Position Stand. 1990. The recommended quantity and quality of exercise for developing and maintaining cardiorespiratory and muscular fitness, and flexibility in healthy adults. *Med Sci Sports Exerc.* 22: 265–74.

18. Bo et al. 2005. Lower urinary tract symptoms.

19. Kraemer, W. J., Adams, K., Cafarelli, E., Dudley, G. A., Dooly, C., Feigenbaum, M. S., Fleck, S. J., Franklin, B., Fry, A. C., et al. 2002. Progression models in resistance training for healthy adults. *Med Sci Sports Exerc.* 34: 364–80.

20. DiNubile, N. A., Patrick, W. 2005. *FrameWork*. Emmaus, PA: Rodale.

21. Sapsford, R., Hodges, P. W. 2001. Contraction of the pelvic floor muscles during abdominal manoeuvres. *Arch Phys Med Rehabil.* 82: 1081-88.

22. Waterstone, M., Wolfe, C., Hooper, R., Bewley, S. 2003. Postnatal morbidity after childbirth and severe obstetric morbidity. *BJOG* 110: 128-33.

23. O'Connell, H. E., Sanjeevan, K. V., Hutson, J. M. 2005. Anatomy of the clitoris. *J Urol.* 174 (1): 1189-95.

24. Chalker, R. 2000. *The Clitoral Truth: The Secret World at Your Fingertip*. New York: Seven Stories Press.

25. Berman, L. 2010. *It's Not Him, It's You!: How to Take Charge of Your Life and Create the Love and Intimacy You Deserve*. New York: DK Publishing.

26. Bo, K. 2004. Pelvic floor muscle training.

27. Ibid.

Chapter 8. Additional Conservative Treatments

1. Agency for Health Care Policy and Research. 1996. Overview: Urinary Incontinence in Adults, Clinical Practice Guideline Update. www.ahrq.gov/clinic/uiover vw.htm (accessed 5/26/11).

2. Bump, R. C., Norton, P. A. 1998. Epidemiology and natural history of pelvic floor dysfunction. *Obstet Gynecol Clinics North America* 4: 723-46.

3. Mayo Clinic Staff. 2010. Kegel Exercises: A How-to Guide for Women. *Mayo Foundation for Medical Education and Research*. www.mayoclinic.com/health/kegel -exercises/WO00119 (accessed 5/26/11).

4. Medical News Today. 2006. Kegel Exercises Reduce Urinary Incontinence in Women, Study Confirms. www.medicalnewstoday.com/articles/37110.php (accessed 5/26/11).

5. Connell, K., Guess, M. K., La Combe, J., Wang, A., Powers, K., Lazarou, G., Mikhail, M. 2005. Evaluation of the role of pudendal nerve integrity in female sexual function using noninvasive techniques. *Am J Obstet Gynecol.* 192 (5): 1712-17.

6. Davila, G. W., Ghoniem, G. M., Wexner, S. D., eds. 2010. *Pelvic Floor Dysfunction: A Multidisciplinary Approach*. London: Springer.

7. Simon, Harvey, M.D., reviewer. 2006. Incontinence Medications. *Health Central*. www.healthcentral.com/incontinence/treatment-000050_13-145.html (accessed 5/26/11).

8. Gillenwater, J. Y. 1991. *Adult and Pediatric Urology*. St. Louis: Mosby Year Book.

9. Raz, R., Stamm, W. E. 1993. A controlled trial of intravaginal estriol in postmenopausal women with recurrent urinary tract infections. *N Engl J Med.* 329:753-56.

10. Mayo Clinic Staff. 2009. Bladder Control Problems: Medications for Treating Urinary Incontinence. www.mayoclinic.com/health/bladder-control-problems/ w000123 (accessed 5/26/11).

11. Speroff, L., Fritz, M. 2004. *Clinical Gynecologic Endocrinology and Infertility*. Philadelphia: Lippincott Williams and Wilkins.

12. Diokno, A. C., Appell, R. A., Sand, P. K., Dmochowski, R. R., Gburek, B. M., Klimberg, I. W., Kell, S. H., OPERA Study Group. 2003. Prospective, randomized, double-blind study of the efficacy and tolerability of the extended-release formulations of oxybutynin and tolterodine for overactive bladder: Results of the OPERA trial. *Mayo Clin Proc.* 78: 687-95.

13. Simon, Harvey, M.D., reviewer. 2011. Stress Incontinence. *New York Times* http://health.nytimes.com/health/guides/disease/stress-incontinence/medications .html (accessed 5/26/11).

14. Nathorst-Böös, J., Wiklund, I., Mattsson, L. A., Sandin, K., von Schoultz, B. 1993. Is sexual life influenced by transdermal estrogen therapy? A double-blind placebo controlled study in postmenopausal women. *Acta Obstet Gynecol Scand.* 72: 656-60.

15. American Academy of Family Physicians. 2009. Bladder Training for Urinary Incontinence. www.familydoctor.org/online/famdocen/home/seniors/common-older/ 798.html (accessed 5/26/11).

16. Bump, R. C., McClish, D. M. 1992. Cigarette smoking and urinary incontinence in women. *Am J Obstet Gynecol.* 167 (5): 1214-18.

17. Simon, H. 2011. Stress Incontinence.

18. Denson, M., Houser, E. 2006. Improving the symptoms and quality of life of patients with overactive bladder and urinary incontinence. The Urology Team, PA.

19. Ibid.

20. Ibid.

21. Subak, L. L., Whitcomb, E., Shen, H., Saxton, J., Vittinghoff, E., Brown, J. 2005. Weight loss: A novel and effective treatment for urinary incontinence. *J Urol.* 174 (1): 190-95.

22. Schmidt, Jasmine. 2007. Acupuncture and Tai Chi as Incontinence Treatments. IncontinenceNetwork.com.www.healthcentral.com/incontinence/c/45/10980/tai-chi (accessed 5/26/11).

23. National Institute for Health and Clinical Excellence. 2011. Percutaneous Posterior Tibial Nerve Stimulation for Overactive Bladder Syndrome. Guidance issued, IPG362. www.nice.org.uk/ip822 (accessed 9/21/2011).

24. Regence (Oregon and Utah). 2011. Surgery Section—Posterior Tibial Nerve Stimulation for Voiding Dysfunction (Policy No. 154). http://blue.regence.com/trg medpol/surgery/sur154.html (accessed 9/23/2011).

25. National Collaborating Centre for Women's and Children's Health. 2006. Urinary Incontinence: The Management of Urinary Incontinence in Women. www.guide line.gov/content.aspx?id=9926 (accessed 9/20/2011).

26. Regence. 2011. Surgery Section.

27. Ibid.

28. Ibid.

29. Ibid.

30. Ibid.

31. National Collaborating Centre for Women's and Children's Health. 2006. Urinary Incontinence.

32. Burrows, L. J., Shaw, H. 2008. Contemporary management of pelvic organ prolapse. *Menopause Management* (Sept.-Oct.): 23-30.

33. Clemons, J. L., Aguilar, V. C., Tillinghast, T. A., Jackson, N. D., Myers, D. L. 2004. Patient satisfaction and changes in prolapse and urinary symptoms in women who were fitted successfully with a pessary for pelvic organ prolapse. *Am J Obstet Gynecol.* 190 (4): 1025-29.

34. Burrows and Shaw. 2008. Contemporary management.

35. Santucci, R. A., Payne, C. K., Saigal, C. S., Urologic Diseases in America Project. 2008. Office dilation of the female urethra: A quality of care problem in the field of urology. *J. Urol.* 180 (50): 2068-75.

Chapter 9. Surgical Solutions

1. National Institutes of Health, Medline Plus. 2009. Urinary Incontinence—Retropubic Suspension. www.nm.nih.gov/medlineplus/ency/article/007374.htm (accessed 5/26/11).

2. Denson, M., Houser, E. 2006. Treatment plan for pelvic floor prolapse. The Urology Team, PA.

3. Deval, B., Ramsay, I. 2005. Transobturator tape: A new method of treatment of female stress urinary incontinence? *Obstetrician and Gynaecologist* 7: 192-94. Campbell, M. F. 2002. Urologic surgery. In *Campbell's Urology*, 8th ed. Philadelphia: W. B. Saunders.

4. Lobel, B. A., Manunta, A., Rodriguez, A. 2001. The management of female stress urinary incontinence using the sling procedure. *BJU Int.* 88 (8): 832-39. Richter, H. R., Varner, R. E., Sanders, E., Holley, R. L., Northen, A., Cliver, S. P. 2001. Effects of pubovaginal sling procedure on patients with urethral hypermobility and intrinsic sphincter deficiency: Would they do it again? *Am J Obstet Gynecol.* 184 (2): 14-19.

5. National Institutes of Health. 2009. Urinary Incontinence. Chapple, C. R. 2007. Retropubic suspension surgery for incontinence in women. In *Campbell-Walsh Urology*, 9th ed., vol. 3. Philadelphia: Saunders Elsevier.

6. Nikolavsky, D., Flynn, B., Gonzalez, C. 2002. Pelvic slings for stress urinary incontinence: Are all created equal? *J Urol.* 167: 608-12.

7. Porena, M., Costantini, E., Frea, B., Giannantoni, A., Ranzoni, S., Mearini, L., Bini, V., Kocjancic, E. 2007. Tension-free vaginal tape versus transobturator tape as surgery for stress urinary incontinence: Results of a multicentre randomised trial. *Eur Urol.* 52 (5): 1481-90.

8. Nikolavsky et al. 2002. Pelvic slings.

9. Deole, N., Kaufmann, A., Arunkalaivanan, A. 2011. Evaluation of safety and efficacy of single-incision mid-urethral short tape procedure (MiniArc tape) for stress urinary incontinence under local anaesthesia. *Int Urogynecol J Pelvic Floor Dysfunct.* 22 (3): 335-39.

10. Nikolavsky et al. 2002. Pelvic slings. Schierlitz, L., Dwyer, P. L., Rosamilia, A., Murray, C., Thomas, E., De Souza, A., Lim, Y. N., Hiscock, R. 2008. Effectiveness of tension-free vaginal tape compared with transobturator tape in women with stress urinary incontinence and intrinsic sphincter deficiency: A randomized controlled trial. *Obstet Gynecol.* 112 (6): 1253–61.

11. Kennelly, M. J., Moore, R., Nguyen, J. N., Lukban, J. C., Siegel, S. 2010. Prospective evaluation of a single incision sling for stress urinary incontinence. *J Urol.* 184 (2): 604–609. Nikolavsky et al. 2002. Pelvic slings.

12. Olsson, I., Kroon, U. 1999. A three-year postoperative evaluation of tension-free vaginal tape. *Gynecol Obstet Invest.* 48 (4): 267–69. Jeffry, L., Deval, B., Birsan, A., Soriano, D., Daraï, E. 2001. Objective and subjective cure rates after tension-free vaginal tape for treatment of urinary incontinence. *Urology* 58 (5): 702–706.

13. National Institute for Clinical Excellence. 2003. Guidance on the use of tension-free vaginal tape (Gynecare TVT) for stress incontinence. *Technology Appraisal Guidance* 56: 15.

14. Mukherjee, K., Constantine, G. 2001. Urinary stress incontinence in obese women: Tension-free vaginal tape is the answer. *BJU Int.* 88 (9): 881–83.

15. Ulmsten, U., Falconer, C., Johnson, P., Jomaa, M., Lannér, L., Nilsson, C. G., Olsson, I. 1998. A multi-centre study of tension-free vaginal tape (TVT) for surgical treatment of stress urinary incontinence. *Int Urogynecol J.* 9: 210–13.

16. Lo, T. S., Huang, H. J., Chang, C. L., Wong, S. Y., Horng, S. G., Liang, C. C. 2002. Use of intravenous anaesthesia for tension-free vaginal tape therapy in elderly women with genuine stress incontinence. *Urology* 59 (3): 349–53.

17. Stanford, E., Levy, B., Rosenblatt, P. 2005. The use of mesh in pelvic reconstructive surgery. *OBG Management: A Supplement* S81.

18. Nilsson, C. G., Falconer, C., Rezapour, M. 2004. Seven-year follow-up of the tension-free vaginal tape procedure for treatment of urinary incontinence. *Obstet Gynecol.* 104: 1259–62.

19. Meschia, M., Pifarotti, P., Bernasconi, F., Guercio, E., Maffiolini, M., Magatti, F., Spreafico, L. 2001. Tension-free vaginal tape: Analysis of outcomes and complications in 404 stress incontinent women. *Int Urogynecol J Pelvic Floor Dysfunct.* 12 (suppl. 2): S24–27. Ulmsten et al. 1998. A multi-centre study of tension-free vaginal tape. Wang, A. C., Lo, T. S. 1998. Tension-free vaginal tape: A minimally invasive solution to stress urinary incontinence in women. *J Reprod Med.* 43: 429–34.

20. Nilsson, C. G., Kuuva, N., Falconer, C., Rezapour, M., Ulmsten, U. 2001. Long-term results of the tension-free vaginal tape (TVT) procedure for surgical treatment of female stress urinary incontinence. *Int Urogynecol J Pelvic Floor Dysfunct.* 12 (suppl. 2): S5–8. Rezapour, M., Falconer, C., Ulmsten, U. 2001. Tension-free vaginal tape (TVT) in stress incontinent women with intrinsic sphincter deficiency (ISD)—a long-term follow-up. *Int Urogynecol J Pelvic Floor Dysfunct.* 12 (suppl. 2): S12–14.

21. Jomaa, M. 2003. A seven-year follow-up of tension-free vaginal tape (TVT) for

surgical treatment of female stress urinary incontinence under local anaesthesia. *Int Urogynecol J.* 14 (suppl. 1): S69-70.

22. Kuo, H. C. 2001. The surgical results of the pubovaginal sling procedure using polypropylene mesh for stress urinary incontinence. *BJU International* 88 (9): 884-88.

23. Vasavada, S. P. 2011. Pubovaginal Sling. *eMedicine from WebMD.* http://emedi cine.medscape.com/article/447951-print (accessed 5/26/11). Woodruff, A. J., Cole, E. E., Dmochowski, R. R., Scarpero, H. M., Beckman, E. N., Winters, J. C. 2008. Histologic comparison of pubovaginal sling graft materials: A comparative study. *Urology* 72 (1): 85-89.

24. Falton, B. 2009. Is there any evidence to advocate SUI prevention in continent women undergoing prolapse repair? An overview. *Int Urogynecol J Pelvic Floor Dysfunct.* 20 (2): 235-45.

25. Miklos, J. R., Kohli, N. 2000. Laparoscopic paravaginal repair plus Burch colposuspension: Review and descriptive technique. *Urology* 56 (suppl. 6A): 64-69.

26. Brubaker, L., Cundiff, G. W., Fine, P., Nygaard, I., Richter, H. E., Visco, A. G., Zyczynski, H., Brown, M. B., Weber, A. M., Pelvic Floor Disorders Network. 2006. Abdominal sacrocolpopexy with Burch colposuspension to reduce urinary stress incontinence. *N Engl J Med.* 354: 1557-66.

27. Chapple, C. R. 2007. Retropubic suspension surgery.

28. Milani, R., Scalambrino, S., Quadri, G., Algeri, M., Marchesin, R. 1985. Marshall-Marchetti-Krantz procedure and Burch colposuspension in the surgical treatment of female urinary incontinence. *BJOG* 92: 1050-53.

29. Woodruff, A. J., Roth, C. C., Winters, J. C. 2007. Abdominal sacral colpopexy: Surgical pearls and outcomes. *Curr Urol Rep.* 8 (5): 399-404. Ostergard, D. R. 2007. *Ostergard's Urogynecology and Pelvic Floor Dysfunction.* Philadelphia: Lippincott Williams and Wilkins.

30. Kohli, N., Sze, E. H., Roat, T. W., Karram, M. M. 1996. Incidence of recurrent cystocele after anterior colporrhaphy with and without concomitant transvaginal needle suspension. *Am J Obstet Gynecol.* 175: 1476-82.

31. Lentz, G. M. 2007. Anatomic defects of the abdominal wall and pelvic floor. In *Comprehensive Gynecology*, 5th ed. Philadelphia: Mosby Elsevier.

32. Raz, S., Little, N. A, Juma, S., Sussman, E. M. 1991. Repair of severe anterior vaginal wall prolapse (grade IV cystourethrocele). *J Urol.* 146: 988-92. De Tayrac, R., Deffieux, X., Gervaise, A., Chauveaud-Lambling, A., Fernandez, H. 2006. Long-term anatomical and functional assessment of trans-vaginal cystocele repair using a tension-free polypropylene mesh. *Int Urogynecol J Pelvic Floor Dysfunct.* 17 (5): 483-88.

33. Zimmern, P. E., Leach, G. E., Ganabathi, K. 1993. The urological aspects of vaginal wall prolapse, pt. II: Surgical techniques, complications, and results. *AUA Update Series* 12 (26): 202-207.

34. Kohli, N., Miklos, J. R. 2003. Dermal graft-augmented rectocele repair. *Int Urogynecol J.* 14: 146-49.

35. Yamana, T., Takahashi, T., Iwadare, J. 2006. Clinical and physiologic outcomes after transvaginal rectocele repair. *Dis Colon Rectum* 49 (5): 661-67.

36. Haase, P., Skivsted, L. 1988. Influence of operations for stress incontinence and/or genital des census on sexual life. *Acta Obstet Gynecol Scand.* 67: 659.

37. Tarnay, C. M. 2007. Pelvic organ prolapse. In *Current Diagnosis and Treatment Obstetrics and Gynecology*, 10th ed. New York: McGraw-Hill Medical.

38. Chou, Q., Weber, A. M., Piedmonte, M. R. 2000. Clinical presentation of enterocele. *Obstet Gynecol.* 96 (4): 599-603.

39. Raz, S., Nitti, V. W., Bregg, K. J. 1993. Transvaginal repair of enterocele. *J Urol.* 149: 724-30.

40. Tulikangas, P. K., Piedmonte, M. R., Weber, A. M. 2001. Functional and anatomic follow-up of enterocele repairs. *Obstet Gynecol.* 98 (2): 265-68.

41. Cespedes, R. D., Cross, C. A., McGuire, E. J. 1998. Pelvic prolapse: Diagnosing and treating cystoceles, rectoceles, and enteroceles. *Medscape Women's Health* 3 (4): 4.

42. Begley, J. S., Kupferman, S. P., Kuznetsov, D. D., Kobashi, K. C., Govier, F. E., McGonigle, K. F., Muntz, H. G. 2005. Incidence and management of abdominal sacrocolpopexy mesh erosions. *Am J Obstet Gynecol.* 192: 1956-62.

43. Maher, C. F., Qatawneh, A. M., Dwyer, P. L., Carey, M. P., Cornish, A., Schluter, P. J. 2004. Abdominal sacral colpopexy or vaginal sacrospinous colpopexy for vaginal vault prolapse: a prospective randomized study. *Am J Obstet Gynecol.* 190: 20-26.

44. Zucchi, A., Lazzeri, M., Porena, M., Mearini, L., Costantini, E. 2010. Uterus preservation in pelvic organ prolapse surgery. *Nature Reviews Urology* 7:626-33.

45. Dietz, V., van der Vaart, C., van der Graaf, Y., Heintz, P., Schraffordt Koops, S. 2010. One-year follow-up after sacrospinous hysteropexy and vaginal hysterectomy for uterine descent: A randomized study. *Int Urogynecol J.* 21 (2): 209. Lin, L., Ho, M., Haessler, A., Betson, L., Alinsod, R., Liu, C., Bhatia, N. 2005. A review of laparoscopic uterine suspension procedures for uterine preservation. *Curr Opin Obstet Gynecol.* 17 (5): 541-46.

46. Lentz. 2007. Anatomic defects.

47. Ibid.

48. Siegel, S. W., Catanzaro, F., Dijkema, H. E., Elhilali, M. M., Fowler, C. J., Gajewski, J. B., Hassouna, M. M., Janknegt, R. A., Jonas, U., van Kerrebroeck, P. E., Lycklama à Nijeholt, A. A., Oleson, K. A., Schmidt, R. A. 2000. Long-term results of a multicenter study on sacral nerve stimulation for treatment of urinary urge incontinence, urgency-frequency, and retention. *Urology* 56 (suppl. 6A): 87-91.

49. Amundsen, C. L., Romero, A. A., Jamison, M. G., Webster, G. D. 2005. Sacral neuromodulation for intractable urge incontinence: Are there factors associated with cure? *Urology* 66 (4): 363.

50. Van Kerrebroeck, P., van Voskuilen, A. C., Heesakkers, J. P., Lycklama à Nijeholt, A. A., Siegel, S., Jonas, U., Fowler, C. J., Fall, M., Gajewski, J. B., Hassouna, M. M., Cappellano, F., Elhilali, M. M., Milam, D. F., Das, A. K., Dijkema, H. E., van den

Hombergh, U. 2007. Results of sacral neuromodulation therapy for urinary voiding dysfunctions: Outcomes of a prospective, worldwide clinic study. *J Urol.* 178: 2029-34.

51. Jonas, U., Fowler, C. J., Chancellor, M. B., Elhilali, M. M., Fall, M., Gajewski, J. B., Grünewald, V., Hassouna, M. M., Hombergh, U., Janknegt, R., van Kerrebroeck, P. E., Lycklama à Nijeholt, A. A., Siegel, S. W., Schmidt, R. A. 2001. Efficacy of sacral nerve stimulation for urinary retention: Results 18 months after implantation. *J Urol.* 165: 15-19. Sievert, K. D., Nagele, U., Pannek, J., Engeler, D., Kuczyk, M., Stenzl, A. 2007. Subcutaneous tunneling of the temporary testing electrode significantly improves the success rate of subchronic sacral nerve modulation (SNM). *World J Urol.* 25: 607-12.

Index

acidic foods, 28, 41, 51, 137-38

acupuncture, 128, 140–41; for constipation, 141; effectiveness of, 141; for mixed urinary incontinence, 62; for stress urinary incontinence, 17, 26, 29; for urge urinary incontinence, 47, 52

Agency for Healthcare Research and Quality (formerly Agency for Health Care Policy and Research), 22, 43, 46, 127

alcohol intake, 29, 32, 137, 138

American Academy of Family Physicians, 17, 135, 175

American Association of Sexuality Educators, Counselors and Therapists, 175

American College of Obstetricians and Gynecologists, 175

American Physical Therapy Association, 176

American Urogynecologic Society, 27, 49

American Urological Association Foundation, 176

amitriptyline, 27, 50, 132

anatomy, pelvic, 7–12

anesthesia, 146, 149; for Burch procedure, 160; for cystocele repair, 164; for enterocele repair, 168; for Marshall-Marchetti-Krantz procedure, 162; for prolapse surgery, 76; for pubovaginal sling procedure, 158; for rectocele repair, 166; for sacral colpopexy, 170; for sacral neuromodulation, 173; for tension-free vaginal tape procedure, 155; for transobturator tape procedure, 151

antibiotics, before rectocele repair, 166

antimuscarinic drugs: formulations of, 49, 131; for mixed urinary incontinence, 28, 55; side effects of, 49, 131–32; for stress urinary incontinence, 27, 28, 131; for urge urinary incontinence, 28, 49, 50, 133

antispasmodic drugs, 49, 50

anus, 8, 9

arylalkylamines in diet, 137, 139

fesoterodine, 28, 49, 131
fiber, dietary, 32, 33, 55, 75, 139
fistulas, 45, 150, 163
flavoxate, 50
fluid intake, 6, 33, 136–37, 138; amount
of, 51, 137; for dry mouth, 131; keeping diary of, 24; timing of, 29, 52, 135,
136–37
food. *See* diet

Gelnique, 49
Gittes procedure, 156

health insurance, 14
hernia, 66. *See also* pelvic organ
prolapse
hyoscyamine sulfate, 50
hysterectomy, 76, 146, 172; combined
with other surgeries, 151, 166, 170;
pelvic organ prolapse after, 70, 167,
172

imipramine, 27, 50, 132
International Continence Society, 36, 57
intra-abdominal pressure, 9, 18, 55, 57,
110, 114, 151, 154, 157, 161
intrinsic sphincter deficiency (ISD), 5,
7, 150, 157

juices, citric, 32, 51, 75, 138

Kegel exercises, 129; for decreased
sexual sensation, 78; effectiveness of,
89–90, 126, 130; for pelvic organ prolapse, 65; for stress urinary inconti-

nence, 13–15, 47, 130; for urge urinary
incontinence, 44, 47–48, 51. *See also*
pelvic floor muscle retraining
kidneys, 11

laparoscopic surgery: Burch procedure, 147, 159–60, 161; hysterectomy,
172; Marshall-Marchetti-Krantz procedure, 162; sacral colpopexy, 170,
171; uterine suspension procedures,
172
laughter, urine leakage with, 2, 6, 15, 16,
18, 34, 41, 47, 55
lifting: after surgery, 148; urine leakage
with, 6, 15, 57, 66, 72, 73, 74, 100, 110,
114, 119, 151, 154
low-back pressure or pain, 2, 6, 63, 65,
70, 168, 170

magnetic resonance imaging (MRI), 72
Marshall-Marchetti-Krantz procedure,
30, 145, 159, 161–63; candidates for,
161; description of, 161; indications
for, 161; invasiveness of, 162; performance of, 162; risks of, 150; success
rates for, 147, 162–63
Mayo Clinic, 72, 130, 132
medical history, 22, 44–45, 61, 64,
71–72, 85
medication history, 22, 24, 25, 45, 73, 85
medications, 126–27, 128, 130–34; constipation due to, 33, 49, 55, 148; cost
of, 16; for decreased sexual sensation,
85, 87, 130, 133, 134; dry mouth due
to, 33, 49, 50, 52, 55, 131, 132; effec-

tiveness of, 134; for mixed urinary incontinence, 54, 61, 62, 126, 130, 133; for overactive bladder/urge urinary incontinence, 2, 32-33, 34, 42, 44, 46, 47, 49-50, 130, 133; for overflow incontinence, 7; postoperative, 148; resuming after surgery, 148-49; for stress urinary incontinence, 14, 17, 25, 26, 27-28, 130, 131-32; urge urinary incontinence due to, 40, 41, 43, 75

MedlinePlus, 176

menopause, 5, 6, 31, 43; estrogen after, 87, 132, 133; muscle loss after, 86; pelvic organ prolapse after, 70, 71; sexual sensation after, 82, 83, 86, 87, 133

mesh, synthetic: in cystocele repair, 147, 164-65; in enterocele repair, 169; erosion or infection of, 149, 156, 158, 163; in prolapse surgery, 76, 163; in pubovaginal sling procedure, 147, 158, 161; in rectocele repair, 166; in tension-free vaginal tape procedure, 153, 155-56; in transobturator tape procedure, 14, 30, 151, 152

mixed urinary incontinence, 2, 4, 5, 54-62; causes of, 58; conservative treatment of, 62, 126; costs of, 60; cure for, 60-61; definition of, 57; diagnosis of, 59, 61; medications for, 54, 61, 62, 126, 130, 133; prevalence of, 57-58; risk factors for, 59; seeking help for, 56-57, 59-60; story of recovery from, 54-55; surgery for, 62, 153; symptoms of, 4,

6-7, 55-56; talking to doctor about, 61-62; worsening over time, 60

National Association for Continence, 15, 28, 176

National Institute of Clinical Excellence, 153

National Institutes of Health, 28, 29, 49, 146, 176

National Kidney and Urologic Diseases Clearinghouse, 176

National Overactive Bladder Evaluation (NOBLE) study, 37

nicotine, 28, 136. *See also* smoking

nocturia, 1, 6, 24, 32, 34, 36, 40, 41, 92

North American Menopause Society, 176

obturator fossa, 152, 155

obturator internus muscle, 152

orgasm, 3, 6, 79, 81, 82, 83, 84, 86, 92, 124

Otto, Lesley, 141

overactive bladder/urge urinary incontinence, 1-2, 3, 5, 31-53; causes of, 38-40; conservative treatment of, 34, 44, 47-53, 141-42; costs of, 43; cure for, 43-44; description of, 36-37; diagnosis of, 44-46; medications for, 2, 32-33, 34, 42, 44, 46, 47, 49-50, 130, 133; pelvic floor muscle retraining for, 32, 47-49, 92; percutaneous tibial nerve stimulation for, 47, 52-53, 141-42; postoperative onset of, 149; prevalence of, 2, 33, 34, 37; risk

71-72; after hysterectomy, 70, 167, 172; intrinsic sphincter deficiency and, 5; pelvic floor muscle retraining for, 65-66, 74, 92; postoperative recurrence of, 73, 165, 167, 169; prevalence of, 3, 67; risk factors for, 66, 70-71; seeking help for, 71; story of recovery from, 63-64; stress urinary incontinence and, 19; symptoms of, 65, 67, 70, 72-73; talking to doctor about, 72-73; vaginal pessary for, 7, 71, 74, 75, 128, 142-44, 168, 170; worsening over time, 71

pelvic organ prolapse surgeries, 3, 64, 67, 71, 75-76, 88, 163-72; cystocele repair, 163-65; enterocele repair, 167-69; rectocele repair, 165-67; risks of, 163; sacral colpopexy, 169-71

percutaneous tibial nerve stimulation, 47, 52-53, 141-42

perineum, 9, 95, 166, 167

pessary, vaginal, 7, 71, 74, 75, 128, 142-44, 168, 170

physical therapy, 128; for decreased sexual sensation, 3, 78, 84, 86; for mixed urinary incontinence, 54-55; for pelvic organ prolapse, 74; for stress urinary incontinence, 14, 17, 22, 27; for urge urinary incontinence, 2, 32, 48

Pilates, 78, 120

post-void residual, 23, 45, 61

Prelief, 137

procidentia, 66, 67. *See also* uterine prolapse

Program to Reduce Incontinence by Diet and Exercise (PRIDE), 52

pubic bone, 8

pubococcygeus ("love") muscle, 82

pubovaginal sling procedures, 30, 145, 156-58; candidates for, 157; description of, 157; indications for, 156; invasiveness of, 157-58; older types of, 156-57; performance of, 158; risks of, 150; success rates for, 147, 158

quality of life, 2, 4, 5, 16, 17, 33, 42, 56, 60, 142

Raz procedure, 156

rectocele, 5, 66-67, 165

rectocele repair, 76, 146, 165-67; candidates for, 165; description of, 165-66; invasiveness of, 166; performance of, 166-67; success rates for, 147, 167

rectum, 8, 9

relaxation techniques, 14

resources, 175-77

retropubic space, 150

sacral colpopexy, 146, 169-71; Burch procedure and, 161; candidates for, 170; description of, 170; indications for, 169; invasiveness of, 170; performance of, 170-71; robotic-assisted, 171; success rates for, 147, 171

sacral neuromodulation, 7, 52-53, 62, 142, 146, 147, 172-74; candidates for, 173; description of, 173; indications for, 172-73; invasiveness of, 173; performance of, 173; success rates for, 147, 174

screening, 22-23, 44-45, 61

sexual activity: benefits of good sex, 80; cystocele and, 164; pain during, 6, 65, 70, 78, 163, 164, 167; rectocele repair and, 167; after surgery, 148; vaginal pessary and, 75, 144

Sexuality Information and Education Council of the United States, 177

sexual sensation, decreased, 3, 4, 77-88; cause of, 81-82; conservative treatment of, 83, 85-87; cure for, 83; definition of, 81; diagnosis of, 84; indications of, 82-83; medications for, 85, 87, 130, 133, 134; pelvic floor muscle retraining for, 3, 77-78, 85-87, 92-93; pelvic floor strength and, 9, 77, 79-80, 81-82; prevalence of, 81, 130; risk factors for, 83; seeking help for, 83-84; story of recovery from, 77-78; surgery for, 88; symptoms of, 6-7; worsening over time, 83

smoking: bladder cancer and, 136; cessation of, 28, 44, 66, 74, 92, 127, 135, 136; decreased sexual sensation and, 83, 87; pelvic organ prolapse and, 70, 72; stress urinary incontinence and, 19, 136; urge urinary incontinence and, 41, 51

sneezing, urine leakage with, 6, 9, 13, 14, 15, 18, 19, 55, 57, 59, 110, 125, 153

Society for Sex Therapy and Research, 177

Society for the Scientific Study of Sexuality, 177

solifenacin, 28, 49, 131

Stamey procedure, 156

stress urinary incontinence, 1, 3, 5, 13-30; bladder in, 19, 20-21; cause of, 1, 13-15, 18-19; conservative treatment of, 17, 23, 26-29; cost of, 16-17, 21; cure for, 22-24; definition of, 18; diagnosis of, 22-24; medications for, 14, 17, 25, 26, 27-28, 130, 131-32; pelvic floor muscle retraining for, 13-15, 26-27, 91-92, 129, 130; postoperative recurrence of, 149, 162-63; prevalence of, 1, 15, 18; risk factors for, 19; seeking help for, 18, 20-22; story of recovery from, 13-15; surgery for, 14-15, 17, 29-30, 147, 150-63; symptoms of, 4, 6-7, 24; talking to doctor about, 24-25; urge urinary incontinence and (see mixed urinary incontinence); worsening over time, 22

sugarless gum/candy, 51, 55, 131, 137

surgical procedures, 145-74; anesthesia for, 146, 149, 155; Burch procedure, 30, 145, 159-61; general considerations for, 149-50; hysterectomy, 70, 76, 146, 151, 166, 167, 170, 172; for intrinsic sphincter deficiency, 7; Marshall-Marchetti-Krantz procedure, 30, 145, 159, 161-63; for mixed urinary incontinence, 62, 153; for overactive bladder/urge urinary incontinence, 34, 53, 147, 153, 172-74; for pelvic organ prolapse, 3, 64, 67, 71, 75-76, 88, 163-72; postoperative guidelines after, 148-49; pubovaginal sling, 30, 145, 156-58; risks of, 146, 149; sacral neuromodulation, 7,

52-53, 62, 142, 146, 147, 172-74; for stress urinary incontinence, 14-15, 17, 29-30, 147, 150-63; success rates for, 147; tension-free vaginal tape, 145, 149, 153-56; transobturator tape, 14-15, 30, 145, 149, 150-53

tension-free vaginal tape procedure, 30, 145, 153-56; candidates for, 154; description of, 154; indications for, 153-54; invasiveness of, 154-55; performance of, 155-56; risks of, 149; success rates for, 147, 156
timed voiding, 51, 135-36
tolterodine, 28, 49, 131
transobturator tape procedure, 14-15, 30, 145, 150-53; candidates for, 150; description of, 151; indications for, 150; invasiveness of, 151-52; performance of, 152-53; risks of, 149; single-incision, 145, 147, 151, 152-53; success rates for, 147, 153; triple-incision, 151, 152, 153
transversus abdominis muscle, 115
treatments. *See* conservative treatments; pelvic floor muscle retraining; surgical procedures
tricyclic medications: side effects of, 50, 132; for stress urinary incontinence, 27, 132; for urge urinary incontinence, 49, 50, 133
trospium chloride, 49, 131

ultrasound, 72
ureters, 11

urethra, 8, 9, 12, 150; dilation of, 144; hypermobility of, 150, 153, 157, 159, 161
urethral bulking agents, 5
urge urinary incontinence. *See* overactive bladder/urge urinary incontinence
urinalysis, 23, 45, 61
urinary catheterization, 7; postoperative, 149-50, 155
urinary incontinence: costs of, 16-17, 21, 43, 60; mixed, 2, 4, 5, 54-62; overflow, 7; postoperative recurrence of, 149, 162-63; prevalence of, 15, 18; stress, 1, 3, 13-30; urge, 1-2, 3, 31-53
urinary retention, postoperative, 149, 154
urinary system, 10-12
urinary tract infection, 16, 23, 41, 43, 132, 164; postoperative, 150
urination, normal, 12
urine acidity, 28, 137-38
urodynamic testing, 23-24, 46, 58, 61, 72
urogynecologist, 22, 25, 27, 44, 48, 64, 66, 128
urologist, 22, 25, 27, 32-33, 44, 48, 53, 65, 70, 76, 84, 85, 99, 128, 141, 144
UroToday, 177
uterine prolapse, 66, 67; hysterectomy for, 172; uterine suspension procedures for, 146, 171-72

vagina, 8, 9
vaginal pessaries, 7, 71, 74, 75, 128, 142-44, 168, 170